Mike —
Best wishes
always & —
Keep winning!

Ken Roberts

A Runner's Guide

Russ Ebbets

Copyright 2019 by Russ Ebbets
The book author retains sole copyright to
his contributions to this book.

Published 2019.
Printed in the United States of America.
All rights reserved.

No portion of this book may be reproduced, stored in a retrieval system, or transmitted in any form or by any means—electronic, mechanical, photocopy, recording, scanning, or other—except for brief quotations in critical reviews or articles, without the prior written permission of the author.

ISBN 978-1-950647-15-6

Disclaimer

The content provided in this book, including text, treatments, dosages, charts, profiles, graphics, images and advice are for informational purposes only and do not constitute the providing of healthcare advice. The information provided is not intended to be a substitute for independent professional healthcare judgment, diagnosis, or treatment.

The content is not intended to establish a standard of care to be followed by a user of the book. You understand and acknowledge that one should always seek the advice of a physician or other qualified health provider with any questions or concerns regarding one's health. You also understand and acknowledge that you should never disregard or delay seeking professional advice relating to treatment or standard of care because of information contained in this book.

Healthcare information changes constantly. Therefore, the information in this book should not be considered current, complete or exhaustive, nor should you rely on such information to recommend a course of treatment for you or any other individual. Reliance on any information provided in this book is solely at your own risk.

Publishng assistance by BookCrafters, Parker, Colorado.
www.bookcrafters.net

Dedication

To Frank DeMasi
Coach
Colleague
Friend
Catch you on the other side.

Other books by Russ Ebbets

Supernova
High Peaks Str8 Maps
Time and Chance

Acknowledgements

There are always many people to thank with the publishing of a book. While the end product may be a labor of love for the author it is often the "other" individuals whose help ultimately makes the book happen. Special thanks go to Mark Mindel, Tim St. Lawrence and Harry Marra for their critiques and kind words. And finally, to Joan Parsnick for her artistic touch.

Invocation

For we run by faith,
not by sight.
- 2 Corinthians 5:7

Night is longer than day
for those who dream.
Day is longer than night
for those who make
their dreams come true.
- Jack Kerouac, author of *On The Road*

Only the fit are fearless.
– Percy Wells Cerutty

Table of Contents

Introduction..1
Only the Fit are Fearless...5
Race Starting..9
Into My Office...14
The 4 Levels of Sport..22
11 Keys to a Successful Running Program...............27
100 Meter Rehab..36
Acid-Base..41
Anatomical Adaptation..48
Anatomy Trains..53
The Foot Drills..58
Barefoot Madness..63
Children Running: Can v. Should..............................67
Core Stability..73
Destination Runs..81
Detraining...86
Dynamic Stability...91
Fun—Commitment—Performance...........................98
Hard Level Floors..103
Havana Dreaming...109

A Wrinkle in Time	115
Hittleman's Yoga	124
Hyponatremia	130
Incidental Exercise	136
Linear People	139
Overtraining	143
Plyometrics	149
Pronation and Supination	153
Shin Splints	162
Sports Psychology	166
The Athletic Triage Model	177
Castor Oil	183
The Biomotor Skills	188
The Hamstrings	193
The Neti Pot	200
The Stretching Controversy	204
Think 145	209
Training Theory	213
Competition Travel Tips	220
Vitamin C	225
When I was a Child	230
The 10 Day Rule	234
Training Maxims	238
The Bijou Mile	249

Introduction

It all seemed to get started with a guy named Lutz Dombrowski. He was an East German long jumper who trivia buffs know as the first man to long jump 28'. He did that jump to win the 1980 Moscow Olympics. It is an accomplishment that tends to get lost in the annals of track and field because of Bob Beamon. At the time of Dombrowski's jump Beamon held the world record at 29'2 ½" set 12 years earlier in Mexico City. Details, details.

What fascinated me about Dombrowski was the seeming perfection of his jump. His approach run appeared so symmetric as to border on mechanical. His takeoff and flight were an example of classic hitch-kick form. I was amazed that a human could exhibit such perfection. How did he learn to do this?

That wonder carried over into my graduate studies at Norwich University in Vermont in the fall of 1980. As part of our graduation requirements we had to write a thesis. After several false starts I settled on doing a comparative analysis of the Communist Bloc Olympic development programs and contrasting those with the haphazard American method of developing distance runners. I chose five American distance runners to study: Marty Liquori, Bill Rodgers, Eamonn Coughlin, Mary Decker and Patti

Lyons-Catalano. Granted Coughlin was Irish by birth but I justified his inclusion as his greatest successes came as a product of the American System, such as it is.

The development programs of the scientifically directed Communist Bloc countries proved to be meticulous, methodical and closely monitored. The American System proved to be a haphazard combination of myth and magic and a jumble of ideas that although it produced some stellar results there were few common denominators. There was even less of a pattern for the women—one needs to remember that both Mary Decker and Patti Lyons were the first wave of great American female distance runners. They had no role models to model.

Fast forward to 1983 and I see an ad in *Track and Field News* for a study tour to Moscow, USSR to the Institute of Sport and Physical Culture. It cost $2500. At the time I had $2000 in my bank account. I cleaned out the account and went to Russia.

Ronald Reagan was president. The early 80s was the height of the Cold War. The US had boycotted the 1980 Moscow Olympics. International relations were frosty, to say the least.

We were to fly out of Montreal. I took the bus from Saratoga, NY to Montreal. At the border they took my passport and individually asked each passenger where they were going. When I said Moscow, everything stopped. Next thing I know I'm escorted off the bus, into an interrogation room and getting grilled by three guys in suits. They did not care one iota about Lutz Dombrowski. About 9 million questions later I realize they are trying to figure out if I'm the next Lee Harvey Oswald.

After forty-five minutes I am led back to the bus; the loaded, no A/C bus that has been waiting for me on a hot, humid June afternoon. People were not happy to see me. I am—that guy.

The flight over was long. Moscow airport was dark (to save on electricity). There were troops with machine guns everywhere. The workers in the little souvenir shops did their business calculations with an abacus. How quaint, I thought.

In my coaching career I strove to learn at least one new thing each season. Something that would significantly change how I coached. It seemed like my Soviet classes were teaching me two, three, four or five new things a day! I couldn't write down the stuff fast enough. I felt like my head would explode.

The trip included coaches and educators from across the US and Canada. There was a group of guys who would go on to form the National Strength and Conditioning Association. There was another small group of guys I'll call "The Weider Boys." This was a group of four guys who were principals in Joe Weider's *Muscle and Fitness* empire. One of the women confided in me how uncomfortable this group made her. I understood the gist of her comment but countered with, "If something bad happens—I'm following them." Thinking we'd find out how tough those guys with the machine guns at the airport really were.

The classes ended and we're on the long flight home and one of the Weider Boys was standing alone in the plane's galley. It was Bill Reynolds. He had already established himself with several books on strength development and was a well-know contributor to *Muscle and Fitness*. I asked how he got started in writing.

He was very forthright and over the course of 30 minutes emphasized time and again to—just start doing it. "Get published—anywhere," and then he added, "one thing will lead to another." I returned to my seat and started to make a list.

"Anywhere" turned out to be the *Pace Setter Magazine*, the monthly publication of the Hudson-Mohawk Road Runners Club in upstate New York. I approached Ed Neiles and Joe Hein and pitched my idea for a monthly column on training tips or injury prevention. At the time my road race management company was called On The Road, Inc. We were handling 12-15 events a year. I suggested "On The Road" as a column title figuring to get some monthly publicity.

Joe Hein countered with, "Since you're talking about things other than running—how about calling the column, 'Off The Road'?"

I laughed. It made sense and the name stuck.

Since Ed Neiles I've gone through numerous editors— Liz Mielo, Bill Robinson, Christine Bishop who have all been encouraging and supportive.

To date the body of work of the Off The Road column could be called "eclectic." There have been articles on training and injury prevention but also childhood athletic development, biomechanics, psychology, personal reminisces and even some running fiction with stories from my first novel, *Supernova*.

The essays chosen for this volume are presented in no particular order. I think you'll find the chapters are short 10-minute reads and offer a range of thought-provoking comments, suggestions and advice that can enhance one's athletic participation in general and running in particular creating a safer and more rewarding experience.

Russ Ebbets
July 2019

Only the Fit are Fearless

Some things you never forget. Enough said.

When I was 14-years-old I ordered a book, really a pamphlet, from *Track and Field News* called *Running with Cerutty*. It was only about 28 pages long, there were no pictures and the margins were typed uneven, but the pearls I gleaned from those pages never left me. In the many moves since, I've temporarily misplaced the pamphlet, but I've never forgotten its lessons.

Australian Percy Wells Cerutty was one of distance running's great, charismatic coaches. He'd led a life of quiet desperation until age 40 when a nervous breakdown and subsequent health problems almost led to an early death. Fortunately, the spark refused to die, and he spent the remainder of his life extolling the virtues of his sport, a healthy lifestyle and his philosophies in general. He was also one to freely chastise any and all detractors. Opinionated, well-read and always willing to address any audience he made for many a lively interview.

During one nationally televised interview the commentator made a remark Cerutty found particularly insulting. Cerutty reached over the podium and punched the commentator right in the nose! How different would be our lives had Muhammad Ali been so brash.

Cerutty's philosophy was an outgrowth of the Stoic philosophy. Stoics lived an austere lifestyle, showed little emotion and hardened themselves to both pain and pleasure. Cerutty was an unforgiving taskmaster. He challenged his athletes both mentally and physically. The results included Olympic medals and world records.

As Cerutty's fame spread, boxers, soccer players and other athletes journeyed to his training camp at Portsea, Australia to learn his teachings, eat his meals and run his sand hill. The cornerstone of Cerutty's physical training regimen was an 80m sand hill that led from the beach to his camp.

When I started coaching, I used to take the team from Schenectady to a sand hill in Saratoga behind Skidmore College. It made for a long practice. One day while driving on Route 155 I noticed a large sand hill off Kings Road. Upon exploration I found the challenge I had dreamed about as a 14-year-old.

In 10 years of coaching "The Pine Bush" was as much a part of my team's training regimen as was a 400m track. Throughout the fall we'd make weekly trips to the hill. The runners were never late to leave—we didn't wait for the reluctant. Those who cared knew if you were going to be good the Pine Bush was going to make you good.

We ran the hill with three rules: 1. No talking, 2. No throwing sand, 3. Keep moving. The rules were so simple that the uninitiated would laugh. Then, knowing what they knew, the older runners would laugh. Our practice ritual called for us to kneel at the foot of the hill (once you were dirty you didn't worry about getting dirty), stand, give a Zen yell and attack.

For even the most talented, five trips up the hill would reduce one to a snail's pace. Various techniques evolved.

In the step pattern one used the same footprints again and again. It made for a neat and orderly workout. The pioneers broke new ground each trip up. Finally, the "reverts," those that reverted to all fours, crawled up the hill like a child or animal. We moved in silence.

Aside from the fact that this was an enjoyable workout and always well attended there were several training benefits that justified the dirty sox and grit we swallowed. The soft, giving nature of the sand while providing tremendous resistance to forward movement was very forgiving to the foot and ankle. By not giving one a solid base to push off the runners were required to improve their balance and use only actions that led to forward movement. The thighs were forced to drive with each step. At the end of an 8-minute run they would be rock solid.

Cardiovascularly heart rates quickly climbed to 150+. The thing that was great about the hill was that the rate could be maintained without requiring one to bang out a mile and a half at 80% effort. This strengthened the legs and reduced the pounding at the same time. The final quality the hill taught was to be relentless. There was always one more step, one more trip, we never gave up, we kept moving. A freshman once told me that the greatest thing about the Pine Bush was that it made the races seem easy.

For those so inclined the hill we ran is at the intersection of Route 155 and Kings Road. The hill has an old, rusty water tank on the top. I figure that over the years we probably put close to a million footsteps on the hill, although you'd never know it. Each week the wind and the weather gave us a clean slate to work with. Be advised that this workout is not for the faint of heart. Wear old shoes or your new shoes will be old shoes. We always ran time segments of

8-12 minutes. Timing individual runs gets too frustrating. Practice being relentless.

When you are done take one last trip up the hill to look at all your footwork. Looking up and out you'll get a great view of the Helderbergs. For those so inclined you might want to take a minute to commune with old Percy. Only the fit are fearless—Herb Elliot lived and ran by those words. His credits include a 1500m gold at the Rome Olympics, world records in the mile and 1500m and the singular distinction of never having lost a mile/1500m race in his life. Never.

Race Starting

All races begin with a start, yet it is a skill few practice with any great seriousness. Awareness and focus can be two simple actions that get one off "on the right foot" and make for a more successful race effort.

Starting is an aggressive act. One goes from zero to race speed in seconds, through force of will. Also included in the mix of starting are the early stages of the race course that need to be scouted out. Of note are any terrain changes, turns or bottlenecks that can present a tactical advantage or disadvantage depending on how they are approached.

Track racing and in particular, indoor track racing present unique challenges. With 10, 12 or 15 runners vying for pole position into the first turn attempts at early placing can be critical, especially in shorter races like the 600m or 800m.

One of the last races I ran was an indoor 800m at West Point. The meet was put on by the old Metropolitan Athletics Congress (MAC). The meets routinely drew talent levels that ranged from Olympian to no. I was scheduled to race the third heat of three.

On paper one needed a qualifying time of 2:04 or better to enter. In reality, if one stood upright, could fog a mirror and had the $10 entry fee you were in. The third heat was a collection of humanity akin to the Walmart of racing. There were contenders and pretenders. As I scanned my competition, I realized there were guys there who couldn't run a 2:04 if they were in free fall. I distinctly remember lamenting—so this is what it has become?

With such a diverse talent pool and a particularly large field (there were at least 15 runners) I ran through several race scenarios and the options they presented. There would be a crush at the start with all the guys good for at least 50m, then there would be the slow death as one dying runner after another clogged up the track. This would lead to bumping and shoving and almost certainly somebody taking a dive or getting spiked. I resolved to get off the line quick and leave the pack behind to devour itself.

Two of the competitors immediately stood out. The Headband was a chunky guy, maybe 5'8" wearing striped knee sox and trainers. He seemed nervous. I chalked him up as a rookie. The second guy had to be at least 6'8", maybe even 6'9". He was the tallest runner I had ever seen. His most distinguishing characteristic was his neck. He had a neck like a giraffe. Once again, I thought—so this is what it has become?

I pulled starting position #2. As we approached the start line, I could see Headband was going to be in lane 3 and Giraffe in lane 4. If those guys beat me to the corner, my race was over.

In the moment before the gun Headband stood distractedly looking left and right, not sure what was going to happen next. He toed the line with his left foot. This gave me my opening. As I stood in the set position, I brought both my arms in front of me. In that split second of hold I moved my right hand toward the Headband's thigh. With the gunshot I pushed his thigh down holding his foot on the track as I broke for the corner.

In theory my creating a moment's hesitation by the Headband was to give me that precious moment to break on top and avoid the crush of the pack. In theory.

I did not see what happened, only heard. It seems that the Headband lost his balance and with his first step veered right. He crashed into Giraffe on his immediate right. Giraffe in turn veered right and proceeded to fall. Now a 6'8" person who falls, falls in stages. As it happened Giraffe took down five guys with him. As I sped away I heard a jumble of runners' curses and crowd laughter. I knew there would be no recall, after all, this was the third heat. And, this is what it had become.

In the end I finished second. I jogged away from the finish line endeavoring to avoid any finger pointing. I stopped to catch my breath behind the bleachers. Almost instantly the guys from my team came over to congratulate me on my finish, and on my start. One guy summed it up, "Coach, when are you going to teach us how to do that?"

The importance of a race's start is inversely proportional to the distance run. I'll give you a second to reread that sentence. Think about the 100m—the start is critical. Think marathon—the start—not so much.

This is not to dismiss the import of the race start in road races as some of the same fundamental principles apply. Listed below are simple suggestions to keep one's thoughts focused on starting efforts and productive starts.

Identify the Starter—Who is the starter? Where does he or she stand? What commands will be used? Does the starter have a set cadence? Or do they vary their cadence from race to race? Can you watch (and listen) to the starter start other races?

The 1st Step—You toe the line with your lead leg. When the gun goes off—which leg moves first? You have a choice. With the "jab step" the lead leg moves first and you push with your back leg. This is more for a quick indoor track start with many runners in a confined space. Taking a "full stride" by driving the back leg forward is more for cross country or road races that allow for a slightly more relaxed start.

5 Quick Steps—Commit to getting off the line quickly. Five quick steps will get you into the flow of things and one can shift to smooth, quick running strides.

The 1st Turn/Bottlenecks—In a track race, runners break for the pole or inside lane. They are supposed to have a "full running stride" before they do this. It is a violation that always happens and is never called. "Set yourself up for the turn," means make some space for yourself. In road or cross-country races "bottlenecks" are narrow areas of a course that funnel runners. The leaders run unencumbered while the pack gets jostled with stutter steps and jerky running efforts. One should review course bottlenecks beforehand and "set yourself up for the turns" so they can be negotiated smoothly, especially if they are at the early stages of a race when the running pack is still crowded.

Incidental contact—Congestion breeds contact. You might get bumped or pushed. It happens. Accept it and move on. A shove or an elbow are different. Better to forget and move on than try to retaliate. Let the officials do their job.

The Rolling or European Start—This is a track start where the runners use a 2-3 step jog up to the line, hold the set position for a moment and then the gun fires. One must firmly hold the set position as there is a tendency to let momentum continue with the forward lean and create a false start. If your race schedule uses this type of start it behooves you to practice it so the mechanics of the "approach and hold" at the line can be done under control.

The Final Thought—I always trained my runners to think "I am strong, fast and confident" in the moment before the gun shot. This tiny affirmation was used to get them off on the "right" foot, literally and figuratively. And with the gun shot they were ready to race.

A journey of 1000 miles begins with a single step.
                    -Lao Tzu

All races begin with a start. In the shorter races the importance of the start can be critical. The start is a chance to focus one's attention to the task at hand. While starting can be dismissed as a trivial part of the larger race if the first step is a "good" step it can have a domino effect that can build confidence throughout the race. Starting then becomes a skill worth practicing and perfecting.

Into My Office...

A long jumper, a javelin thrower and a coach walk into my office...there should be a joke there, but all I've got is my own little version of Ripley's *Believe it or Not!*

The door to my office at Union was a funnel for a parade of alumni, prospects and suspects that all came with a story to tell in exchange for a moment of my time.

The "Marathoner from Miami" was a kid who wanted to come to college to run the marathon. He already had two under his belt with a PR of 3:06. Frank Shorter was his idol and he made it clear he was going to run the marathon.

I told him the marathon wasn't a college event and that there was strong evidence that running a marathon before physical maturity could hinder athletic development.

"But," his mother added, "my son is a marathoner." It sounded more like a learning disability than a mark of distinction. I was getting nowhere with this pair. I thanked them for making the visit, they left and I dropped the athletic questionnaire in the waste basket.

In the early 80s track on TV was a more regular event. One indoor season produced a series of great mile races between Eamonn Coughlan and Steve Scott. Coughlan's clever tactics produced three great wins that highlighted the indoor season and inspired countless people. "I saw the milers on TV Saturday," began the Pit, "it looks pretty easy, it looks like fun," then he dropped the clincher, "I think I can beat them."

The Pit had black hair, stood about 5'10" and was a fat 170 pounds. The Pit couldn't beat an egg. But what I remember most about the Pit was his eyes. There was a complete vacancy to his stare. He spoke like a drone. There was an uneasy feeling in my stomach. I had heard enough.

I wrote down directions for his physical, practice times and told him to show up when he's been cleared to run. I never saw him again but for the longest time I found myself checking the rooftops for snipers.

It seems "The Miler" was making a career out of college. He would surface every few years take a few courses and then disappear. All the while he'd tell anyone who would listen that he'd run a sub-four minute mile. The problem was no one ever saw him run a step. His previous incarnation was during NCAA Champ Kevin Scheuer's era. Mention this guy to Kevin and he'll spit.

But there was a flip side too. Stan Gasorowski coached at Albany High. One day he gave me a call. "I gotta guy you gotta see..." he began. Periodically I'd sneak one of the top local kids into the Field House to train. "He's a long jumper." I'm thinking Stan's got a kid doing 21'-22'.

"Russ, I know this is going to sound strange but," I'd known Stan for over a decade. He is a solid, no BS guy. "Russ, the guy jumped 26'4" in our pit the other day."

Downhill? Wind aided? Twenty-six feet is still twenty-six feet. I paused a moment. What could I say? Then Stan added, very sheepishly, "Russ, he really jumped 27'4" but if I tell you that I'm afraid that you'll think I'm crazy."

I was trying to process this. "Stan, do you realize what

you are saying?" And before he could answer I added, "That is what Carl Lewis is jumping."

All Stan could say was, "I know." And then he added that 27'4" would be the fourth longest jump in the world last year. He had looked it up in *Track and Field News*.

I told Stan I'd like to meet the guy.

The guy was named Mike Fields. He looked like Willie Banks. He came to the Field House, warmed up and jumped. He ran down the runway with an arm action that was too high, steps that were too long and he jumped 25'6" with a 10-step approach. He said his foot hurt. He didn't want to jump again. I saw what I needed to see.

This guy was more than a diamond in the rough. This guy was history, as in "make history." I looked at Stan and said, "We gotta talk."

Fields was interested in college. He'd jumped 21' in high school, grew six inches since graduation three years ago and wanted to know if I could help him.

I wondered where he would fit in. Fields had his own concerns. He wore a gold neck chain that was thicker than a finger. I wondered more. Fields was a professional gambler. In his own brilliance he'd learned how to write a tip sheet for the California horse tracks which he sent daily over the wire to racetracks in California. Gambling and the NCAA don't mix.

Nonetheless word got out. Florida State called, then Texas and UCLA. The questions were always the same, "Did you see…?" or "Is this guy for real?" All I could say was what I saw. The guy jumped 25' and change on a 10-step approach. Even on a bad day that is an NCAA Division 1 All-American. Fields never pursued his talent. I still wonder.

And there were always the calls out of the blue regarding using the track, getting into a meet or finding a competition. Gary Cudmore of Amsterdam HS called, said he had a foreign exchange student and could this student see me?

The javelin is not a regularly contested event in New York State high schools. The kid showed up with his host mother. The mother did the talking, the kid only spoke broken English. It was quickly apparent that all the mother knew about the javelin was that it was thrown. I explained the NYSHS situation, mentioned some clinics Tommi might attend and told her I would make a call on their behalf to Kevin McGill, one of the top throw experts in America, then at Columbia University.

"By the way, how far does Tommi throw?" The mother didn't know. She asked Tommi. He pulled a thin, glossy covered magazine from his duffle bag. His picture was on the cover, he stood at the center of a podium, arms raised and a gold medal around his neck. The caption was in a foreign language I couldn't read but I did notice the "73m" in the title.

Seventy-three meters. It took a minute for me to translate the metric into English. My hammer thrower was throwing 60 meters which was about 190', a meter is 10% longer than a yard...I ran the numbers through my head and figured this kid was throwing close to 240'. That was close to the US national high school record.

I called McGill. I said, "Kevin, you are not going to believe this..." Every fall Iona College held clinics and competitions for the throwers. We arranged for Tommi to make the trip down. He set the clinic on its ear.

McGill still talks about Tommi Viskari. The perfect form, the powerful arm, the blast off the right foot. The kid was videotaped like a movie star. Later that fall Tommi set the US National High School record for the international weight javelin that still stands. You can look it up. His name is on the same list with Jim Ryun, Rudy Chapa, Gerry Lindgren and Renaldo Nehemiah. Tommi Viskari, Amsterdam, NY, 241'11". (Editor's note—Viskari's record was broken in 2010 by Sam Crouser from Gresham, Oregon)

But the man I remember most was Paul Sweet. Tall and almost gaunt Paul entered my office with a regal carriage that belied his 85+ years of age. I had no idea who he was. I had never heard of him.

Paul introduced himself and asked if I had the time to talk a few minutes. We talked. He was the track coach for the University of New Hampshire for over 60 years. He'd recently retired and was now living in Scotia, NY. Towards the end of the conversation he invited me to his house for dinner. A free meal is a free meal. I accepted.

That three-hour visit has become one of the most fascinating evenings of my life. Initially we spoke about how training has changed. The useful "old methods" were reviewed and the new innovations that have revolutionized the sport were discussed at length. Then he got out the scrapbooks.

Paul had scrapbooks dating from the 1920s. His UNH teams had upwards of 120 members. He pointed with his finger and named runner after runner as if he'd coached them yesterday.

Of particular note was an athlete named Morcom. Boo Morcom and another teammate once won the IC4A Track Championships by themselves. I remembered reading about this two man "team" in Ripley's *Believe it or Not*. Paul provided the details.

Paul also coached Jeff Bannister, one of the top US decathletes in the late 60s. For some reason a picture from *Track and Field News* of Bannister (about 6'6") towering over Bennett (about 5'8") has always stuck in my mind. I asked Paul what he did when he was an athlete. He had a scrapbook for that too.

Paul ran for the University of Illinois. He had a picture of a relay team, all smiles, standing with a coach, all hands on a baton. He told me his coach's name was Harry Gill. It didn't register for a second, then it did.

"Harry Gill of Gill Hurdles?"

He smiled and said yes. The Gill Equipment Company had been one of the major suppliers of track and field equipment in America since the 1920s. He turned the page.

He told me, "This was my best day," and pointed to a yellowed slip of newsprint with the title, 'Illinois Quartet Sets World Record in Relay.' I read on with great interest.

At the Drake Relays Paul had anchored the University of Illinois 4x110 relay to a world record. I couldn't believe it.

"Notre Dame was there," he said, "guess who was their coach?"

I had no idea. I thought a moment and still had no idea. I threw out the only name I could think of, Knute Rockne.

"You're right."

This was getting weird. He asked if I'd finished reading the article. I read on. After setting the world record in the 4x110 Paul and his teammates came back and set the collegiate and American record in the 4x220, missing the world record by 1/10th second. Paul anchored.

Paul was scheduled to run the anchor leg on the 4x440 but strained his Achilles tendon and was replaced by a runner named Fitch.

"Do you know who he was?"

I had no idea, not even a guess.

"Did you see *Chariots of Fire*?"

I had, but I still made no connections. Paul told me

that Horatio Fitch had gotten second to Eric Liddell, the Scotsman in the 400m at the 1924 Paris Olympics.

Paul told me that in the "old days" one couldn't coach and compete at the same time. That was considered professional. He had gotten married; a family was on the way and he'd been offered the coaching position at New Hampshire. A decision was made.

He never said what I thought, but the hint that things would have been different in Paris hung heavily in the next moment's silence.

Paul stood straight against the indignities of old age with 60 years of scrapbooks and the memories they generated. I stood there thinking about Frost's "The Road Not Taken" and marveled at how strange history can be.

Prep Records—Men

Track Events

Event	Mark	Athlete	Location	Date
100	10.13	Derrick Florence (Ball, Galveston, Tx)	Towson, Md	6/28/86
200	20.13	Roy Martin (Roosevelt, Dallas, Tx)	Austin, Tex	5/11/85
	20.13	Roy Martin (Roosevelt, Dallas, Tx)	Indianapolis, Ind	6/16/85
400	44.69	Darrell Robinson (Wilson, Tacoma, Wa)	Indianapolis, Ind	7/24/82
800	1:46.45	Michael Granville (Bell Gardens, Ca)	Norwalk, Calif	5/31/96
1000	2:25.5	Tom Carroll (Fordham Prep, Bronx, NY)	Koblenz, Ger	8/10/57
1500	3:39.0	Jim Ryun (East, Wichita, Ks)	New Brunswick, NJ	6/28/64
Mile	3:55.3	Jim Ryun (East, Wichita, Ks)	San Diego, Calif	6/27/65
2000	5:23.3	Eric Hulst (Laguna Beach, Ca)	Norwalk, Calif	5/28/76
	5:23.30	Michael O'Connor (St John, West Islip, NY)	Uniondale, NY	6/17/86
3000	8:05.8	John Trautmann (Monroe-Woodbury, Central Valley, NY)	Philadelphia, Pa	4/25/86
2 Miles	8:36.3	Jeff Nelson (Burbank, Ca)	Westwood, Calif	5/ 8/79
2000St	5:43.9	Steve Guerrini (Santa Rosa, Ca)	Santa Rosa, Calif	4/27/91
3000St	8:50.1	Jeff Hess (South, Eugene, Or)	Eugene, Ore	6/ 2/79
5000	13:44.0	Gerry Lindgren (Rogers, Spokane, Wa)	Compton, Calif	6/ 5/64
10,000	28:32.7	Rudy Chapa (Hammond, In)	Des Moines, Ia	4/24/76
Mar	2:23:47	Mitch Kingery (San Carlos, Ca)	Burlingame, Calif	2/11/73
(aided)	2:23:05'	Clancy Devery (South, Salem, Or)	Seaside, Ore	2/26/77

Hurdle Events

Event	Mark	Athlete	Location	Date
110H(39")	13.30	Chris Nelloms (Dunbar, Dayton, Oh)	Dayton, Oh	5/26/90
	13.22y	Arthur Blake (Haines City, Fl)	Winter Park, Fla	5/11/84
	12.9y	Renaldo Nehemiah (Scotch Plains-Fanwood, SP, NJ)	Jamaica, NY	5/30/77
110H(42")	13.83	Glenn Terry (Sycamore, Cincinnati, Oh)	Columbus, Oh	6/11/89
	13.5	Renaldo Nehemiah (Scotch Plains-Fanwood, SP, NJ)	Richmond, Va	7/ 2/77
300H	35.32	George Porter (Cabrillo, Lompoc, Ca)	Walnut, Calif	5/25/85
400H	50.02	Patrick Mann (Gar-Field, Woodbridge, Va)	Los Angeles, Calif	6/24/84
	49.8(A)	Bob Bornkessel (Shawnee Miss N, Overland Pk, Ks)	Echo Summit, Calif	8/31/68

Jumping Events

Event	Mark		Athlete	Location	Date
HJ	2.29	7-6	Dothel Edwards (Cedar Shoals, Athens, Ga)	Athens, Ga	7/ 9/83
PV	5.54	18-2	Brandon Richards (San Marcos, Santa Barbara, Ca)	Eugene, Ore	7/11/85
LJ	8.16	26-9¼	Dion Bentley (Penn Hills, Pittsburgh, Pa)	Santa Fe, Arg	6/23/89
TJ	16.39	53-9¼	Brian Tabor (Clarke Central, Athens, Ga)	Columbus, Oh	6/11/89

Throwing Events

Event	Mark		Athlete	Location	Date
SP(hs)	24.78	81-3½	Michael Carter (Jefferson, Dallas, Tx)	Sacramento, Calif	6/16/79
(int)	20.65	67-9	Michael Carter (Jefferson, Dallas, Tx)	Boston, Mass	7/ 4/79
DT(hs)	68.64	225-2	Kamy Keshmiri (Reno, Nv)	Sacramento, Calif	6/13/87
(int)	61.38	201-4	Gregg Hart (Homestead, Ft Wayne, In)	Indianapolis, Ind	7/18/90
HT(hs)	70.68	231-11	Manny Silverio (North Bergen, NJ)	Evanston, Ill	6/12/76
(int)	61.80	202-9	Manny Silverio (North Bergen, NJ)	Providence, RI	8/28/76
JT(hs)	79.20	259-10	Art Skipper (Sandy, Or)	Eugene, Ore	5/28/88
(int)	73.74	241-11	Tommi Viskari' (Amsterdam, NY)	West Point, NY	11/ 3/88
Dec		7359h	Craig Brigham (South, Eugene, Or)	Eugene, Ore	4/22-23/72

(10.9, 6.73/22-1, 14.18/46-6¼, 1.93/6-4, 52.3 [3765],
15.5, 44.16/144-10, 4.43/14-6½, 60.22/197-7, 4:53.0 [3694])

1996 US National High School Records
- Track and Field News Annual Edition

THE 4 LEVELS OF SPORT

Audience questions after a talk often center around "what should I do?" This is difficult unless one establish "where" the athlete is in the grand scheme of sport. The ability to place an athlete greatly helps make some reasonable recommendations as opposed to simply making a blanket statement that may be both age and ability inappropriate.

There are four levels to athletic participation. When one is in the heat of competition this is never a consideration but given a moment of introspection the four levels offer a clear distinction of the possible phases in an athletic career with a direct impact on goals and aspirations.

The first level is the Fundamental Stage. This is one's entry level into sport. Routinely this would begin with simple childhood activities and games in the backyard. With age things may become more organized with youth soccer leagues, little league baseball, biddy basketball

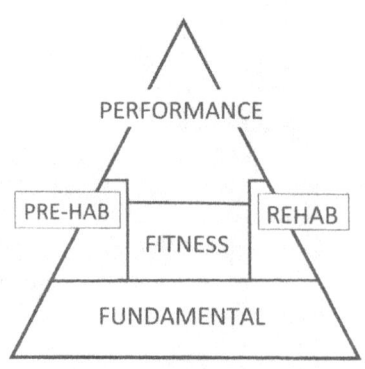

and the like to introduce the mechanics of a sport but also social skills that hopefully morph into early life lessons.

Done properly this Fundamental Stage is critical to an athlete's development. It is here that the patterning of movement skills such as running technique, jumping coordination and throwing mechanics are first introduced and then refined. While technical development should not be the "be all and end all" this input cannot be ignored as "all things only grow once." It is with this thought in mind that the parent, coach or teacher needs to design activities that establish these fundamental movement patterns while at the same time being fun.

Several child sport studies have detailed the fact that the number one reason young athletes quit a sport is due to the sport no longer being fun. This presents a challenge for the parent or coach in that they need to design activities that service both needs. This is a design task that is easier said than done. Nonetheless this delicate balance must be addressed.

A second area of concern is that of growth and development versus training and competition. Youth hockey leagues are notorious for their travel schedules, in some instances rivaling those of collegiate programs. Once again a balance needs to be struck as an overemphasis on the training and competition may stifle the growth and development of the young athlete.

The second stage in sports is that of Fitness. In America it is ironic that this would be the largest area of participation yet we are still struggling with a spiraling obesity problem, the antithesis of fitness. The Fitness Stage includes a period of life where activities are engaged in with the desired effect being some real or perceived benefit.

Weight loss, body shaping, strength or cardiovascular

fitness are all common goals of this stage and can usually be achieved with three to four days a week with some form of regimented activity. Walking, jogging, swimming or cycling would all be common examples of fitness training. Note well that all the above examples are repetitive, possibly mindlessly repetitive and for the most part movement in a linear path. While this may address the cardiovascular component of one's fitness goals it neglects one's overall or multi-lateral development.

Multi-lateral training, recently popularized with the television infomercials such as P-90X address this issue with high intensity multi-directional movements that give not only cardiovascular development but also the overall joint strength and flexibility that more accurately define fitness.

The third stage is that of Performance Based Sport. In this stage competition, winning and achievement of personal goals become paramount. In order to accomplish these goals personal sacrifices, higher degrees of dedication and the limits of mental and physical health are approached.

The Soviet Russians taught that training at the elite levels is not a natural or healthy thing to do for your body. While I initially disagreed with that statement time and training proved to be patient teachers. One need only review the recent news stories on the long-term consequences of the head injuries sustained by football players to see that athletic participation can have its downside. The knees, feet and low backs of runners wear out. Goal oriented performance based training takes its toll on the body.

Success at this stage requires special attention to diet, nutrition, rest and recovery. The attitudes of the fitness stage applied here would reap minimal success. Competition would indicate training regimens of 10-15 hours training per week or more, oftentimes with daily double workouts.

Time in the Performance Stage is counted in dog years. High level participation may last seven to ten or possibly 12 years and then the weight of family commitments, the erosion of skills, accumulation of injuries or the aging process force one to revisit all goals.

The fourth stage actually has two components. Honestly no one gets involved in sport to participate in this stage but it is truly an either/or stage. Either one conscientiously works on the pre-hab (injury prevention activities) or one eventually winds up rehabbing in the breakdown lane.

Pre-hab can be described as anatomical adaptation. This is doing exercises that strengthen or stabilize critical junctions (muscles, ligaments, tendons, joint capsules) in the body. Stabilizing and strengthening these areas help decrease the repetitive stress of training and competition. Long-term there would be a decreased chance of injury and possibly a safer career participation.

Examples of pre-hab work would be core stability work, the foot drills or shoulder stability work. Pre-hab work has been accurately described as invisible training. You can't see the benefits in the mirror but regardless of which level of sport one is participating one would reap the benefits.

Rehabilitation or rehab is the "or" portion of the fourth level. No one signs up for a sport with the goal of becoming hurt, but hurt happens. There is a legion of sports healthcare practitioners who daily care for the poorly conditioned, over trained and under coached masses who fall victim to "too much, too soon" or succumb to the stress of training. Rehab methods range from something as simple as stretching and ice to the more complicated bracing all the way to reconstructive surgery. Equally important are the recovery times that may range from days to weeks to forever. Rehab is never part of the plan, it is the anti-plan.

Athletic participation offers an almost endless opportunity for enjoyment and involvement throughout one's life. In order to make the most of this opportunity it is important one make an honest appraisal of one's current fitness stage and systematically chart a participation plan with a coach, teacher, parent or even a trusted competitor that optimizes the time, effort and energy required of whichever stage one choses to participate in.

11 Keys to a Successful Running Program

Jim Ryun, Tim Danielson and Marty Liquori were the first three high schoolers to run a 4-minute mile. That was in 1965, 1966 and 1967 respectively. It did not happen again until Alan Webb came along in 2001. This Pace Setter *article came out in the early 90s, before Alan Webb emerged. It has always been interesting to run into the coaches who agree and disagree with the points. You can lead a horse to water, but you can't make him drink.*

Distance running is a simple thing. The key to success is putting one foot in front of the other faster than your opponent. The complexity of distance running is its simplicity. As one's involvement increases the nuances of tactics and strategies evolve. Pace, physical preparation, mental focus and a host of other factors combine to spell either success or failure.

I lecture frequently in USA Track and Field's Coaching Education Program. One of my areas is distance training. At the end of the lecture I summarize the presentation with these "11 Keys to a Successful Distance Running Program." These points are the result of personal study, over a decade of coaching and the good fortune to have been blessed with athletes whose faith in the program and motivation towards accomplishment synergistically combined to produce some great results. The simple thing was never simple.

1. **Winning is a learned skill.**

There are many factors that go into the mix of a champion. Some are measurable; speed, strength and endurance while dedication, perseverance and decisiveness are more difficult to quantify.

The Bible says, "Many run the race, but only one will win, run so as to win." One needs to prepare as a champion would. Goal oriented behavior, personal sacrifice, an action oriented mindset, discipline, dedication and a directed willfulness are all "skills" that can be modeled, molded and learned. These are the skills of a champion. Run so as to win.

2. **Run on grass as much as possible.**

Although few of us consider this the days of our lives are numbered. We can influence "the number" by how we live our life. Food selection, personal habits, exercise patterns, environmental and genetic factors all play a role.

It is a logical extension that the number of strides in our competitive running career are also "numbered." Training factors such as shoe selection, workout content, the type of training we do (distance runs, speed work, etc.), coupled with our restoration and regeneration means (flexibility, chiropractic, massage, vitamin supplementation, hydration) are all factors that can influence both the quality and length of a running career.

Another factor is training surface. Running is a "ground contact sport." While our bodies are resilient there is a wear and tear that results from athletic participation. A 150-pound runner places about 35 tons of stress on each leg per mile. That doesn't count the ground reaction forces that can multiply the stress four to seven times.

Hard level surfaces offer little shock absorption and create increased wear and tear. Grass is a more forgiving and less stressful surface. The fact that grass surfaces are slightly uneven enhances one's balance and proprioception playing a secondary role in injury prevention.

3. Limit your runners to three hard efforts per season.

I cannot point to any studies to justify this statement. Experience has taught me this. Even trying to define a "hard effort" can be tough. A race with a long kick, a hot day, a race double, a fast race with a significant time drop—all these factors may make for a hard effort.

Why three hard efforts? My experience has taught me that performance becomes erratic when there are more than three hard efforts per season. There comes to be good races and bad races that are impossible to plan for, which erode confidence and create doubt. Doubt is a cancer of the mind. Race so as to win, with three hard efforts per season.

4. Rest your best people in unimportant races.

Cross-country seasons are generally too long. It is a bad idea to have a high school runner compete more than 11-12 times. The frequent race schedule does not allow for adequate recovery between races. Scheduling commitments may require more racing. Because of this it becomes necessary to periodically and systematically rest runners.

This will be a difficult rule to follow if you are coaching a team with five, seven or ten runners. For a successful season everyone must run every race and do well. It becomes a long season for everyone.

Study the race schedule. What are the dates one can rest people and still do well without a full team effort? Resolve to strategically sit out a runner. This makes rule #3 easier to implement.

This will also develop the leadership by others on the team. They might win or at least they will know that they have produced under pressure. Leadership is a learned skill. See rule #1.

A coach once told me, "You have to let them run all the races—they want to!" Using his logic I countered that we should let them "drink and drive" because they want to. He looked at me like I was an idiot, but he did not have anything else to say. And his teams never beat mine.

5. Avoid the "killer double" of mile-two mile.

Steve Prefontaine has been all but deified since his death. What he could have been is the subject of much speculation. He was the national high school 2-mile record holder with a time of 8:41 and change. That is back-to-back 4:20 miles. As a high schooler he made international teams. He was a man.

Pre ran the killer double three times in high school. He doubled in the 880-mile four more times. He doubled seven times in high school. His other high school marks were a 4:06 mile and a 1:51 half. I don't get what coaches don't see. What is the long-term goal of a coach who lets a kid double seven times in a month?

There is a cumulative stress to distance running. Excessive doubling diverts energy used by the body for growth and development to recovery and survival. The future is spent on the present.

Most coaches are quick to use Pre as a model of performance excellence. Unfortunately for some reason they can't see his high school career as a model for good sense.

6. Never double a steeplechaser—lobby to change the high school distance to 2000m.

The 3000m steeplechase is an exhausting event. It is a commonly held belief that the fatigue created by running the 3000m steeple is equivalent to that of running 10,000m, 6.2 miles. The reason for this is that not only does the steeple require one to run fast but also the immovable barriers and water jump require one to jump and forcefully land over 30x during the course of a race—from one leg to one leg. The race not only exhausts one's aerobic abilities but also one's strength qualities with all the jumping.

Watch most any high school race. For three or four laps the barriers are negotiated smoothly. As fatigue sets in around 4+ laps each barrier is followed by a lengthening recovery period. The strength stores in the athlete are exhausted. The runner struggles to regain momentum for 3-5 seconds and another barrier occurs. The last two laps are done in fits and spurts.

A 2000m race would allow the high schooler to run hard virtually the whole way. Were they to continue at the pace they would produce an excellent 3000m-steeple time. With two years maturity and developmental training they will.

Why never double? If it takes one day to recover for each five minutes raced and the race produces the fatigue associated with a 33-34 minute race (a good high school time) it would take close to a week to recover from one

3000m steeple race. Doubling in the steeple is more of a killer double than the mile-two mile.

7. Limit the number of high school cross-country races to 11-12, in college to 7.

Racing should be used for performance and development. The body will adapt to the stresses placed upon it. There is a cumulative stress to distance running. If the stress is so great or the recovery inadequate energy stores marked for development are shifted towards survival, the result being stunted growth.

The stress accumulates because of inadequate recovery time. This can be shown with numbers. Most high school races are 5000m, with a good male time being 17 minutes, 21+ for females. If it takes the body one day to recover for every five minutes raced it would take a male 3.4 days and a female 4.2 days to recover for each 5000m race.

The average high school program races twice per week beginning in the last week of September and ending about the second week of November. This presents the opportunity to race 15 times using a twice-weekly schedule. The male race schedule barely allows recovery for two races per week and the women are on a negative spiral right from the start. What makes this argument more compelling is that the stress and recovery from hard training days is not even factored in.

All this underscores the importance of rule #4—periodically resting runners from unimportant races. This would allow a 15-date schedule, but not everyone runs 15 dates.

8. Run high school cross-country dual meets at 2.5 miles.

There are several reasons for this. First go back to rule #7. A 2.5-mile race for a male might average 14 minutes to complete requiring 2.8 days of recovery or about 14 hours quicker recovery than a 5000m race. For a female a 17-minute race would require 3.4 days, more than 19 hours quicker or almost a full day less than needed for a 5000m race.

There will also be less stress over the course of a season. Ten races at 14 minutes v. 17 minutes (5000m) for males would mean 30 minutes less race stress on the body over the course of a season. The difference is even greater for women. This produces the equivalent of two fewer races per season.

A second point is speed. The object of racing is to run fast. Any race over three minutes requires endurance. On a championship level speed always wins out over the last 400-800m. Would it not make sense, on the developmental levels, to make speed the preeminent quality to train for?

Once upon a time the course record holder for Van Cortlandt Park at 2.5 miles was a guy named Marty Liquori. He broke four minutes for the mile while still in high school. Jim Ryun holds the high school mile record at 3:55 and change. His high school cross-country races were two miles. Neither ever raced 5000m in high school. The best person still won.

9. Make the home course flat and fast. Train for speed.

Endurance is an easier quality to develop than speed. In fact, physiologists would argue that speed is genetically determined by muscle fiber type, the fast glycolytic fibers.

Nonetheless speed is a technique that can be done right or wrong. And the difference between right and wrong is 10% as it relates to time.

Improving neuromuscular function can influence this 10%—by coordinating the body to quickly execute the desired actions. Part of this coordination is leg turnover rate. Reducing the time of single support ground contact by 1/100th of a second in a 2.5-mile race reduces the total race time by 20 seconds. Reducing the time of ground contact support is a speed action.

Shorter, flatter courses allow for faster running. This allows runners to win with speed. Speed endurance will develop as will pure endurance. Use endurance as a secondary tactic. This needs to be said—all things being equal (which they never are) the faster runner will win, note the word faster.

10. Do not let high school kids race further than 5000m.

There are, but there are few, high school runners who are strong enough to aggressively race 5000m. The rest must submit to the race and become passive in part. Champions are not passive.

We have discussed recovery times—which are more of a factor in a five-mile, ten-mile or longer race. Another thing to consider is leg speed. Long races train slow actions. This is inconsistent with the philosophy of speed. Tactics are generally simpler and take longer to implement. The races unfold slowly; the need to think quickly is less necessary. A long run, a steady state run can have a positive training effect. A long race does little to prepare one for the rigors of a cross-country or a track season.

11. Let frosh be frosh, don't move them up.

I always dressed the freshman team in large t-shirts. They never fit, too big. In the pictures the frosh team looked like hell. One time a mother brought this to my attention, "You bought the wrong shirts," she said. I told her I didn't. I told her that everything I did with the team had a reason. I told her I was encouraging them to grow. That is a true story.

Winning is a learned skill and competition is intimidating. Large invitationals, with the flurry of activity, the colors and sounds can be terrifying to a frosh. Varsity competition will simply overwhelm them. Freshmen need time to get used to this.

A strong developmental program gives the freshman something to grow toward, something to hope for, something to dream about, to develop an expectancy for. Freshmen identify more with their frosh teammates than with seniors. They make plans together and will motivate each other, now and in the future. This develops a sense of cohesiveness and team spirit. Great teams have great spirit.

Let the varsity be a goal. Goal achievement generates excitement. Excitement breeds enthusiasm. Enthusiasm precedes success. Success comes with growth. Encourage them to grow.

Athletic development should be the result of managed control. The coach can control most all the "rules" on the list. Doing enough things right allows great things to happen. Train for speed. Don't over race. Develop the patience to let development come with the turn of a calendar page and not the sweep of a second hand. Winning is a learned skill so run and train and live so as to win.

100 Meter Rehab

"Return to play" from an injury is a difficult decision for the returning athlete and supervising coach. Use of repeat 100m runs can help reintroduce the stresses of running without the risk of a re-injury happening 3 miles from home.

Athletic participation breaks down into one of four areas—fundamental development, physical fitness, performance-based sport and prehab/rehabilitation efforts. The vast, vast majority of athletic people fall into the physical fitness category, probably well over 90%. This participation is for the real and perceived health and lifestyle benefits derived from the routine training regimens.

Performance based sport is where competition is used and the outcomes, wins or loses, personal bests or stellar performances are the preeminent goal. Interesting, or oddly my Russian teachers taught that training at this elite level is not a natural or healthy thing to do for your body.

The fourth category is prehab and rehabilitation. Prehab is a relatively new concept where effort is used to help prevent injuries common to sport. Rehabilitation is the process where an ill or injured person is returned to a previous state of health. Note it is a "process," meaning a progressive, step-by-step means where health, physical fitness or elite performances are hopefully regained.

We all get hurt from time to time. Although as a coach I always was of the opinion that injuries did not have to happen if training was done correctly. A big "if." Injuries still did happen from a slip or trip or some other "accident" that was beyond our control.

Whatever the cause the injured state becomes a starting point from which one must progress back to a state of health that allows one to train and compete at one's pre-injury level.

Classically there are seen to be four stages of rehabilitation: denial, anger, depression, acceptance. The severity of one's injury and one's psychological makeup (read that as stubbornness) all contribute to when and even if one will return to performance training anytime in the near future.

One of the great challenges with injury rehabilitation, particularly for a motivated athlete is their reluctance or inability to take the necessary steps, the rest and recovery and possible therapies to regenerate an injured area. It has often been said that one's greatest strength is one's greatest weakness. The drive and determination one uses to succeed in a competitive situation, the ability to battle the elements, pain and fatigue actually becomes a mindset that is counter productive when it comes to injury rehabilitation.

There are several analogies that can be used to characterize the mindset of the injured and rehabilitating athlete but at their basic level the athlete is doing work that is pain free. That needs to be emphasized—pain free.

The problem comes that this is seen as "babying oneself" and is totally contrary to what has made one successful (one's greatest strength...). But there are two realities here. First, one is no longer in the fitness or performance mode, one is in the rehab mode. Secondly, if one chooses to "gut it out" and limp through the pain you can make an injury last forever—and that is not an exaggeration.

Why is limping, or favoring one body part so dangerous? All movement patterns require their own set of biomechanics. There are healthy biomechanics and inefficient, dangerous biomechanics. When one trains with a limp, favoring one side or the other extra stresses and pressures are placed on the healthy side.

Sooner or later this produces a secondary overuse syndrome somewhere else which if improperly rehabbed can lead to subsequent injuries reverberating back and forth between the legs—an "injury" that lasts forever.

So one has reached the acceptance stage and has chosen any number of sensible rehabilitation methods from bike riding, swimming, weight training, yoga, Somatics, water running or some other treatment that is moving one towards a pain-free state. The opportunity to run looms on the near horizon. Finally, one's advisors (coach, chiropractor, therapist) has given the green light to resume performance training. The new dilemma arises—what is the first step?

What I used very successfully with my athletes was what I called "100 meter rehab." Once they felt they were capable of returning to some type of running I put them on a track and had them run repeat 100-meter runs.

Lest anyone get the wrong idea these were not sprints, they are not even strides or any type of fast runs. It was jogging in a straight line for a predetermined time at an easy pace. It should be added that we had them run on a lane line so that they would run straight.

All the prehab pre-exercise warm-ups would be done—foot drills, some running technique work, calisthenics, in general a good warming up of the body and then the 100m repeats would begin.

No doubt some are saying—how boring that must be, running on a track? For a distance runner? All true, but that is the point. I never wanted the athlete to start back doing anything too difficult.

Besides doing too much there are several other benefits to their 100-meter repeats. A track is flat so the ground contact from stride to stride is consistent. In that many running injuries, particularly for women, are due to lower extremity instability issues, the use of a consistent surface helps decrease this complicating factor.

Other benefits are that the runner runs straight placing even stresses on the legs. This allows one to concentrate on form, good running biomechanics, that need to be consciously reestablished so that they become habitual and ultimately unconsciously produced actions.

It's boring. True, but this is an opportunity to focus on one's mechanics as opposed to "zoning out." The fact that one must stop, turn around and repeat every 100m becomes a not so subtle reminder of what should be the focus of the workout.

Running the 100m does not allow one to run too far or too fast. If something starts to hurt, you are only 100m from home—stop and get some ice. As for the speed issue, speed actions are the only actions of the five biomotor skills (endurance, strength, flexibility, skill and speed) traditionally not addressed in rehab programs. Remember you are rehabbing, not training. There is a critical distinction there.

The first day may entail the warmup, 10 minutes of the repeat 100m runs (or 8-10-12x 100m, if desired) and an easy warm down with stretching, pool therapy or ice.

Slowly over the course of a week one can expand the time of the runs to 20 minutes. Once this becomes "easy" one can add what I called "snake runs," a weaving type run where one zigzags the width of three lanes over the course of 100m. This will develop some additional ankle strength and proprioception further addressing any instability issues.

Once one had progressed 7-10 days without incident the same techniques (100m runs, snake runs) on a soccer or football field can be done. The turf field would be slightly more uneven further challenging and developing one's balance and proprioception.

The final step in this progression is to introduce three-minute runs followed by a one-minute rest. Obviously these will not be on a straight line, but rather a circuitous course is recommended. Over the course of days one can build up to 30 minutes in total running. Once this is achieved pain-free one can safely resume training.

While the causes of one's injury can be multiple and varied rehabilitation needs one's focus and attention. There is a different mindset between the injured rehabilitating athlete and the athlete who uses exercise for either physical fitness or performance.

The use of 100m repeat runs is a safe, simple yet effective means to reintroduce one to the stresses and strains of daily training.

Injury, while certainly not one of the goals of athletic participation is none the less an everlooming reality. It provides one with the opportunity to reevaluate one's goals as to their appropriateness and sensibility. It is a time that can be used wisely and an experience that should make one wiser in terms of preventive care and future training decisions.

Acid-Base

You are what you eat. You hear this all the time. The acid-base qualities of fluids and foods is another perspective that offers some choices for designing a healthy lifestyle and optimizing performance.

Water is the body's solvent. Virtually all the processes of the body need water to happen. Digestion, circulation, elimination are all affected by our water stores and the lack of water or dehydration can have a significant affect on these processes in both the short and long terms.

In the classic book *Your Body's Many Cries for Water* author Batmanhelidj effectively argues that dehydration is at the core of most of the illnesses and diseases generic man succumbs to. To paraphrase Thoreau—most (wo)men lead lives of chronic dehydration.

Maybe the most telling result of this chronic dehydration is that it causes the body to age faster. I need only reference one's 25th high school reunion to make the point. Those "hard livers" who have spent the last 25 years smoking and drinking have paid the price, and they show it.

Water has the unique chemical property of having a neutral pH of seven on a 14-point scale. Most water is at the balance point between an acid (numbers below 7) and a base (numbers above 7). The natural physiological pH for most people's bodily fluids ranges between 7.3—7.4. This is all "nice to know" but what does it mean?

A quick review of Chem 101 is necessary to make the point. The pH of the body refers to the acid-base balance. An equal acid-base balance is 7.0, usually the pH of most water samples. Acidic foods and beverages (with a pH below 7) would include coffee, sodas, sugars, alcohol and most processed foods. Basic or alkaline foods have a pH above 7.0 and would be things like fruits and vegetables and most juices.

One of the problems of the American diet is the prevalence of acid-based foods for the majority of people. Not only do these "foods" fuel the obesity crisis but they create an acidic environment within the body. This acidic environment slows the recovery process and in some cases promotes degenerative diseases such as cancers, heart disease, diabetes and even osteoarthritis with the joints not getting the nutritional support they need for repair.

You are what you eat. Most people get this. Care must be taken to eat a more natural, less processed diet. It is easy to get preachy about this but the importance needs to be underscored. Nothing goes in your mouth by accident. A certain level of mindfulness—staying in the here and now may differentiate healthy choices from simply the easiest choice.

The acid-base balance of the body can even be traced to our breathing patterns. In yogic thought the most important "food" is one's breath. In fact, there is a yogic saying, "He who half breathes, half lives." Improper breathing patterns due to poor posture, spinal scoliosis or nervous tension can have a subtle, yet insidious affect on the acid-base balance and long-term health.

Most know that oxygen is necessary to sustain life. We

get oxygen or O2 when we breathe in. The waste product of respiration is carbon dioxide or CO2. When compared on a molecular level CO2 is considered to be a heavier gas than O2. If you check out the molecular weights on a Periodic Table you can do the math. CO2 has a molecular weight of 28 with O2 weighing in at 16.

Chemically CO2 acts as an acidic gas, O2 is the basic gas. Another fact that most people never consider is that when one breathes in and out the lungs never fully clear, there is always a little gas (CO2) left in the lungs to prevent their collapse. This little extra is called the residual volume and since it is CO2, the heavier gas, it settles in the bottom or lower lobes of the lungs.

For a healthy person this is no big deal. The constant exchange of CO2 and O2 is an unconscious reflex. But for those with compromised lung function due to a long history of smoking, lung cancer or COPD there is an inability of the lungs to expel the CO2 increasing the percent of CO2 in that residual volume and tipping the acid-base balance towards the acidic. This creates a condition called metabolic acidosis and usually forecasts a series of system wide problems past the lung disease.

Somehow the yogis of old figured this out centuries before traditional medicine had advanced to the point where it could diagnose the condition. In yoga there are several recommended "inverted positions" where the practitioner positions the lungs above the head or mouth. The shoulder stand and downward dog are two common examples. (Fig. 1)

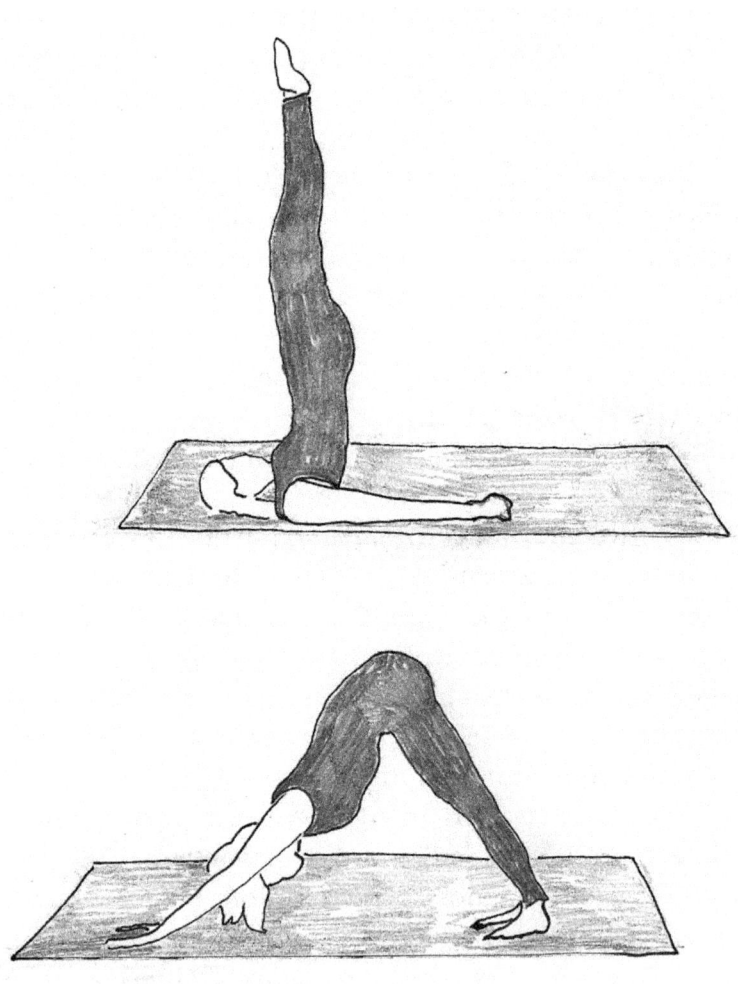

Figure 1. Pictured are the shoulder stand and the "downward dog."
Begin with 15-30 seconds and build to a minute or two.
Make sure your area is obstacle free!

You might think—what does this do? You need to recall that CO_2 is a heavier gas than O_2. Just as gravity affects how an apple falls from a tree the "heavier object," in this case the CO_2, "sinks" towards the lower opening (the mouth) effectively "cleaning out" the residual volume and oxygenating this area.

A final influence on the chemical balance of the body is our thoughts. While I realize this may be a stretch for some it is an accepted fact that thought is the result of a chemical process.

Actually, thought is a biochemical process. You know this. Extreme examples would be getting drunk when the chemical, in this case alcohol, upsets the balance of one's normal thought patterns and subsequent actions. Use of psychedelic drugs such as LSD would be another example. Yet another example would be low oxygen situations experienced by pilots or mountain climbers that can significantly influence thoughts and behaviors.

Note that all these examples happen fairly rapidly, in minutes to hours. But what if there were circumstances that went on for months, years or decades? The changes could be slow and insidious but I think you can see changes would happen and they could be profound.

Sustained emotional states of hate, anger, fear, anxiety, regret, revenge or depression all create chemical reactions to life's stressors. Over the course of time these states not only affect our thought patterns but also how we breathe and even our posture. And if one's posture is altered that will in turn alter breathing patterns which will affect oxygenation. Note the slumped shoulders and forward lean of the depressed person. He who half breathes, half lives and is probably depressed also.

Conversely the person who lives life in the "here and

now" with appreciation, joy for simple things, wonder, thankfulness, optimism, love and charity creates a mental state that promotes health from the inside out. For these people the glass is always half-full, at the very least.

The solutions to maintaining a balanced body pH are fairly simple. Number one recommendation would be to get fresh air on a daily basis. Make it a habit to get outside and take what our grandparents called a "breather" at least twice a day. Breathe deeply, hold that breathe and be thankful you have the opportunity to do so.

Secondly make a consistent effort to drink 8-10 eight-ounce glasses of water on a daily basis. Read that as water, not juice, coffee, tea or some other fluid. Remember you need water to break down the other fluids and foods you ingest.

Thirdly, strive for a water-based diet. Shoot for 80% of the food intake to be as natural as possible. Fruits and vegetables should comprise the majority of this 80%. Try to keep your protein sources of a high quality and if it comes from a box or is highly processed—avoid it.

Mentally strive to maintain a positive mindset. The practice of mindfulness, staying in the "here and now," focusing on the good and being thankful for what you have all create a state that reduces negative stress on the mind and body.

A final check is to monitor one's morning urine on a daily basis. Using acid-base sensitive litmus paper and a few drops of urine one can get a daily check of where body pH is. Acidic morning urine (pH lower than 7) indicates the desired alkaline state in the body. The converse is also true. The "flip" of the pH takes place in the kidneys.

Tested consistently you will come to see that certain foods create certain states, both desired and not desired.

This method is also a valid test for how training and recovery are going. An alkaline morning pH would be a sign of an acidic body indicating that one's recovery from a previous day's workout is not complete or may be the early warning sign of a cold or other illness. Rest, recovery and some vitamin C may be in order.

Most chain drug stores carry the referenced litmus paper or look for MicroEssentials on the Internet. You will want the litmus paper with a pH range of 5.5-8.0 for best results.

You don't hear much about the acid-base balance in the popular press yet but it is knowledge that can be used to make daily training more effective, prevent overtraining, live a healthier life today and even prevent the early aging of the body in the long run.

Anatomical Adaptation

Anatomical adaptation has been called "invisible training" along with such concepts as multi-lateral development, sport psychology and programmed recovery because you cannot "see" the results of countless hours of work. Yet for the performance-based athlete anatomical adaptation is an integral part of a comprehensive training plan.

In the celebrity culture that has evolved in the US one of the preeminent goals of "the American Way" is to always "look good." This runs counter to one of our earliest parental lessons that you can't tell a book by its cover but the reality is that first impressions are lasting and we know we all do it.

There is an application of this faulty thought pattern to sport or at least athletic activities. Bodybuilding is an activity where one endeavors to create a muscular physique that has an aesthetic appeal. This physique is produced through the development of muscle bulk that is more fashion than function. If there is any doubt I would direct you to the Internet to look up "the world's biggest biceps" or "the world's biggest calves" to witness a grotesque display of aesthetics run amuck.

When I studied in the Soviet Union the sports professors scanned our glossy fitness magazines with great incredulity. While there was no doubt some voyeuristic appeal to the telling pictures the question that quickly followed was—why would someone do something like this? What was the function?

What escaped the Russians was that they were evidencing a culture clash of "looking good" versus "being good." For a performance based athlete from a performance based culture the deeper concern lies not in the book's cover but rather the book's content.

We actually have an example of this in running. Were we to poll members of the Hudson Mohawk Road Runners Club as to why they run no doubt the more frequent answers would include the sentiments of "aerobic development" and "cardio-vascular health." These thoughts are an outgrowth of the running revolution of the 80s championed by Kenneth Cooper's Aerobics and the work he pioneered at the Cooper Institute in Texas.

Aerobic training is a paradigm, or thought-belief system that most runners blindly adhere to never considering that there could be another way. To most, to even consider that aerobic development is not the be-all and end-all is heretical, akin to the bumper sticker—God is Dead.

Anatomical adaptation is a concept where the body is trained or prepared in such a way to be able to safely and successfully meet the demands of running or sport in general. Anatomical adaptation is a series of exercises, sport specific, that focus on developing strength and functional integrity of the ligaments, tendons and joint capsules of the body. I'm willing to bet big money that you've never looked in the mirror to secretly admire the development of your ligaments, tendons or joint capsules. At its most basic level anatomical adaptation can be understood as "training to train."

But how does one train these holding elements?

Effectively a ligament or tendon has little to no contractile qualities and any "sense" one has from these tissues is only when they are sprained, overused or otherwise injured. The training of these tissues is not on the radar screen of most runners, particularly those whose sole understanding of training is in the aerobic paradigm.

To train the ligaments and tendons requires one to shift gears and broaden the athletic preparation experience to include strength work and skill development. It requires the paradigm shift.

Before we go on, please understand that I am not discounting the importance and necessity of aerobic development for the runner or endurance athlete. What I am suggesting is that one needs to broaden the understanding of the demands of sport and appreciate what needs to be accomplished for a higher level training to get done.

The body adapts to the stresses placed upon it. To develop ligament and tendon strength and stability one must devise exercises that stress these holding elements.

Strength training is the simplest way. There are several reasons for this. Weight training is the most common form of strength training but here we must clarify that the work required is full body training. Note that you do not need a ton of equipment to do this.

One exercise is to use a 6-10 pound medicine ball. Touch the ball on the ground between the legs and then raise it over your head. This is what is called a multi-link exercise. You are using many, many muscle groups and multiple joint complexes to get this done. What you are accomplishing is to develop strength and coordination of the whole body, not just a specific focus on something like the biceps or quads that one might get by simply doing a bodybuilding exercise.

A second exercise is to consider circuit training. Circuit training is a series of exercises done one after the other. A common pattern is 30-15, 30 seconds of exercise followed by 15 seconds of rest. What exercises are done? The list is almost endless; push-ups, sit-ups, squat thrusts, jumping jacks, short sprints, etc. You are only limited by your imagination. Putting the exercises on index cards, shuffling the cards further allows for an almost endless variety. How many exercises you do is determined by your fitness level. Start with 8-10 stations and as fitness improves go to 15-20.

Circuit training can be done as part of a warm-up or used as conditioning after the main part of a workout is completed. For the endurance athlete circuit training allows for the design of a workout using diverse skills creating a greater skill inventory, strengthening the holding elements of joints that would not normally be addressed with simple linear running work day after day. It also costs very little money and could be done in your cellar or back yard.

A final area of attention is the foot drills. We have frequently talked on this subject before in previous columns. The use of inverted, everted, toe-in/out, heel and toe walking will clarify the nerve pathways to the foot, improve balance and proprioception of the foot, strengthen the ligaments and tendons of the foot and subsequently improve force application. This is a tremendous return for three minutes work. Google "foot drills" if you need more particulars.

For the competitive runner speed qualities are necessary for success. Speed is a function of strength, not one's aerobic base. Certainly aerobic work will constitute the majority of training for the endurance athlete. But a critical component towards increasing both quality and quantity of one's aerobic work will be the attention throughout a training season to focused strength work that will create stronger, more stable holding elements (ligaments and tendons) creating within the body a state we have termed anatomical adaptation.

Anatomy Trains

Traditionally anatomy is taught using a "parts" method of teaching. One body part is learned, and the student moves on to the next body part. But is this the only way? And is this the way we live? Adherents to the Anatomy Trains perspective of the human body would disagree.

The anatomy of the body has been classically taught with a segmental or part by part approach. If we use the arm as an example one would study the biceps, triceps, brachioradialis and deltoid muscles with their circulation, innervation and various attachment sites. Once mastered the student would progress to the next "part" of the body.

While this method has stood the test of time it is flawed in that it does not explain or even address the inter-relatedness and coordination of the body parts, which is how we live.

This becomes problematic on a number of levels. With the classical education teaching the "parts method" there is the natural extension of thought to diagnose in a "parts" way. Shoulder pain, for example, becomes a problem with the shoulder and the shoulder only.

In fact, about two decades ago someone theorized that laterally swaying shoulders in a runner was actually the result of tight hips. The statement was generally ignored if not dismissed outright as nonsense. But right or wrong few took the time to understand how that conclusion was arrived at.

The simple components of our skeletal and muscular system are the muscles, bones, ligaments, tendons and the muscles' fascia. Most people would be familiar with the muscles, bones and ligaments but I'm not sure everyone understands the fascia.

The fascia is a connective tissue that surrounds a muscle. It is a thin, almost transparent tissue that essentially holds the muscle fibers tightly together. It is similar to the cellophane wrapping meat is sold in. Fascia has a contractive quality—it can shorten over time which can affect how a muscle contracts, how a joint works and how a person stands and walks.

The other important thing about fascia is that it comes in sheets, called fascial planes that are connected head to toe. This may seem like a radical statement but only so if human anatomy is seen in the context as a part by part assembly. When the body is viewed holistically it would make sense there is some underlying part to part connection past the skin.

In truth this is not a new concept. Body work specialists who use the Rolfing Technique have used this principle for years to restructure the body by segmentally and in unison manipulate the fascial sheaths allowing the body to assume a posture that is closer to the ideal.

A recent contribution to this body of knowledge is the work of Tom Myers and his book *Anatomy Trains*. What Myers has done is to painstakingly chart out the fascial sheaths that run throughout the body.

He explains his work using railroad analogies. The fascial sheaths are tracks with various joint complexes being junctions. While on the surface these analogies may seem simplistic they adequately represent the fact that the sheaths are in fact linked together throughout the body top to bottom, front to back and with diagonal patterns that cross the body.

But why is this even a concern? This knowledge has clinical implications that help explain certain injuries or injury patterns that would be unsuccessfully treated if one was to simply use a site-specific symptom based approach.

Countless examples abound. You've no doubt heard that fallen arches can cause knee or low back pain. Biomechanically there is the tug of internal rotation that takes place with the pathologically pronated foot but there is also the fascial connection that drags along a joint or in this case several joints to create a structurally unsound posture that can overtime produce the knee or back pain.

Seen in this light one can begin to understand that tight fascia at the hips through its fascial connection to the shoulders causes the trunk to sway laterally as the runner proceeds forward in a true sense struggling against both their physiological limits and a less flexible anatomy as well.

Your mother's admonitions about standing up straight were not only right but also have had lifelong implications. One begins to see that posture, as a component of good health, is really a total body activity.

The problem that civilized man and woman faces, especially in industrialized societies is that our lifestyle promotes poor postures that lead to fascial shortening patterns that lead to excessive wear and tear on joints and their muscular attachments. This combines to lead to early breakdown and injury.

Three quick examples illustrate this point. We all sleep with our feet in a plantar flexed position—toes pointing straight down. This leads to a chronic shortening of the gastrocsoleus complex and the loss of the ankle's ability to dorsiflex. This puts excessive strain on the gastrocsoleus leading to micro-tears, then larger tears, Achilles' tendonitis and calf pulls. If your weak link is below the ankle you get plantar fasciitis. This is all along Myers' posterior longitudinal line.

Many people sit for an occupation. Hip is flexed to 90 degrees and knee is flexed to 90 degrees. This position leads to a chronic shortening of the hamstrings and psoas. Eight hours spent in this position and when one tries to stand up low back stiffness or pain quickly registers. Over the course of time the ligaments of the hip lose the ability to extend the hip and the next thing you know you are walking with the forward lean posture of an elderly person. This is evidence of another of Myers' lines.

Our final example is forward head carriage. Ideally the ear should reside just above the point of the shoulder (the AC joint). When we sit, we tend to hunch over our work, head in front of the shoulder. This does two things—it produces a chronic strain on the muscles of the upper back and leads to a chronically shortened SCM (sternocliedomastoid) or front neck muscles. What further exacerbates this condition is that most people sleep with their head propped up by a big fluffy pillow. This pillow keeps the head flexed for another 6-8 hours.

It is interesting to note that all three of these postures take about 15 years past maturity to slowly develop as problems. At age 35 we start to present with the results of classic overuse syndromes.

So what is the solution? It should be obvious that one needs to incorporate some form of flexibility and strengthening work to counteract the ravages of modern lifestyles, gravity or aging. Yoga, Pilates, T'ai Chi or whatever, there are many disciplines that would do the job. It is important to realize that as we age we become more linear in our activities and that there are significant consequences to this unconscious choice.

I have had the opportunity to work with a number of world class athletes and one point I constantly have to reiterate is that their quest for excellence is also a journey of great specialization and that one happens to the detriment of the other. Well-rounded development needs to be a fundamental concept for both quests and journeys.

The same holds true for the recreational athlete. And it is with visionaries like Tom Myers that one can use his work to broaden horizons and develop deeper appreciation for the demands competitive activities, fitness related pursuits and modern day life stressors have on the body.

The Foot Drills

When I spoke at the High Performance Summit on 'How to Improve Distance Running in the US' for Brooks Johnson in 2005 my opening remarks were, "It has taken me 18 years to get this audience." And then I proceeded to beat home the importance of the foot drills for strengthening the foot, clarifying the neuromuscular pathway from the brain and ultimately improving performance. If you are a visual learner someone from Florida made a nice YouTube video—The Six Foot Drills that also gets the point across.

Over the last decade I have had the good fortune to lecture on track and field and distance running throughout America and the world. The topic of the day could be sports psychology, training theory or biomechanics but I always try to slip in a comment on the importance of the six foot drills. In many instances it may seem totally unrelated but if performance is one's ultimate goal, and if only one thing is remembered from the day's lecture—I hope it is the six foot drills.

I got the idea for the foot drills from my study in East Germany in 1987. Quite honestly there was little value to that study tour. The East Germans seemed confused by our questions and their presentations were disjointed and generally pointless. They did show us one Super 8 film on foot drills for high jumpers. It didn't register at the time.

I've subsequently studied several people's work, including Edgar Cayce, who discussed the benefits and virtues of doing daily foot exercises for prevention of a multitude of foot and leg problems. In 1987 the foot drills were integrated into my team's daily training plan and the grand experiment began.

We did the six foot drills at the start of each practice. Five of the six foot drills are done barefooted or in stocking feet. The distance covered for each drill is about 25 meters. Each drill is done once daily. The walking is done at one's own pace. Total time for the drill with shoes off to shoes on is about four minutes. Pretty simple.

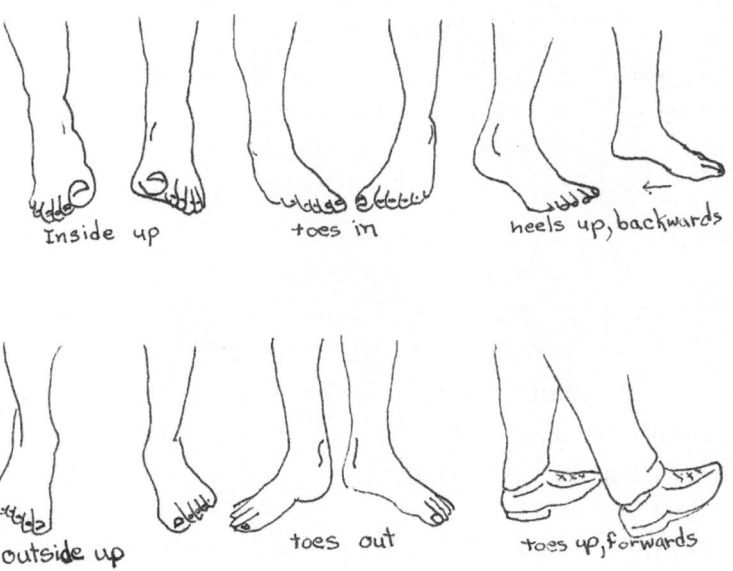

Figure 2. The 6 Foot Drills are done barefooted except for the heel walk. The series can be done in any sequence. L-R, top to bottom – inside up (foot inverted), toes in, heels up backwards toe-walk, outside up (foot everted), toes out à la Charlie Chaplin, toes up heel walk with shoes on.

The six drills, illustrated in Figure 2, are to simply walk on the outside of the foot (invert the foot), walk on the inside of the foot (evert the foot), walk with a toe-in or pigeon-toed gait (adduct the foot), walk with the toes pointing out (à la Charlie Chaplin), walk backwards on the toes (or forefoot) and with the shoe back on, walk on the heels—this protects from bruising the heels.

Done daily these six drills will eliminate shin splints, Achilles' tendonitis, plantar fasciitis, lessen the chance of a severe ankle sprain and virtually all knee problems. The famous Rice Study done in the early 90s found that 79% of running injuries are from the knee down. One of the reasons I had successful teams is that my athletes made it to the competition day healthy and ready to compete. Season after season was completed with virtually no injuries.

It should be noted there are three problems with the foot drills: they are simple, they are easy and they are free. It doesn't involve more than taking off one's shoes and putting one foot in front of the other. But that is easier said than done.

Why do the foot drills work? There is very little muscle in the foot. This presents a problem because most of the balance and proprioception we get comes from our muscles. A second point is that the neuromuscular pathway (the communication line) from the brain to the foot is the longest and slowest in the body. This leads to bad, or at best, poor coordination of the foot. If you doubt that, put a pen between your toes and try to write your name.

The demands of athletic participation, be it running, jumping or quick starts and stops places tremendous stresses on the foot. In fact, the foot must sustain seven times the body's weight with simple running and up to 20x body weight in some jumping activities. Done repeatedly this is how an overuse syndrome such as shin splints, plantar fasciitis or Achilles' tendinitis develops.

By challenging the foot with various gaits one develops a clearer pathway from the foot to the brain. Clearer pathways are faster and more responsive. This gives one better balance and proprioception. Each foot strike becomes more "sure," the foot contacts the ground without a wobble however slight that wobble might be. It is because of this "sure foot strike" that the overuse syndromes (Achilles' tendinitis, plantar fasciitis or shin splints) are eliminated.

It has been said that running is a ground contact sport. It is this repeated micro trauma of ground strike, repeated 1000s of times that can lead to injury. Other factors such as running surfaces and proper shoe selection can influence the incidence of injury. But I will contend with a great deal of assurance, that the six foot drills, done consistently, will have a tremendous positive benefit on one's athletic participation and performance. Applying the simple, easy and free.

The last note. The foot drills will also make you faster. I mentioned the slight "wobble" of each foot strike. More accurately described, a wobble is a lateral, side to side motion. Speed is generally straight ahead. If, on each foot strike there is a wobble or lateral motion before there is forward motion, there is lost time, not much, but some. If one's ground contact time can be reduced 1/100th of a second (it takes 14/100ths of a second to blink the eye) the cumulative effect can drastically improve one's performance.

Consider this—if one takes 50 steps in the 100m, 50x 1/100th = 50/100 seconds or ½ a second. One-half second is the difference between the 9th place spectator and the Olympic Gold Medalist. In the mile this reduced ground contact time translates to an 7-8 second difference and in the 10k it means 40-50 seconds. An improvement made in the blink of an eye, one step at a time. Simple, easy and free.

Barefoot Madness

This June 2012 article sums up the wisdom of the bandwagon effect. Shoe wear is a critical component of athletic success, but it is a strong foot that should benefit from a good shoe, not a weak foot benefitting from a fancy shoe.

If I invited you over for dinner and put a plate of salt in front of you and told you to "dig in" you'd think I'd lost my mind. Salt is a food seasoning. It is meant to enhance the flavor of food, not replace it. Salt is an element of cooking and diet and nutrition, not a meal.

The same is true of barefoot running. Over the last two to three years a fad has surfaced where an appreciation of the role of a "strong foot" has hit the consciousness of the athletic world—and Madison Avenue. Ever in the quest for something new this "minimalist" movement has struck with full force.

Proponents will speak with conviction about how these glorified socks have eliminated their foot and leg problems and rejuvenated their running careers. Given enough time these barefoot zealots will get to the Kenyans and wax poetic about the shoeless culture that has dominated distance running in the world for over four decades.

The problem with these personal testimonies is that they represent the science of one. For a teenager,

20-something, 30-something or a master who was raised in an industrialized nation and spent their life on hard level floors the abrupt change to the minimalist shoe often represents a shock of such magnitude that the ligaments, tendons or muscles of the leg become overwhelmed and breakdown occurs. It is a situation of too much, too soon and injury is the result.

I have become known for touting the foot drills, which are done barefoot on a soft surface. So why would I rail against this minimalist movement which is essentially just an extension of the foot drills?

The problem lies in one's understanding of training. There are training elements and then there are training methods. The foot drills are a training element. Barefoot running is a training element. Interval, repetition or fartlek running would be training methods. It's an example of salt as a seasoning versus salt as a meal.

When a workout is properly designed it should have three components. A warmup, main theme development and a warm down. The 20-30 minute warmup should be used to not only heat up the inner core but this is also an opportunity to sharpen technical movements and skills while the athlete is strong and fresh. Weak links or problem areas can be addressed with specific attention to address the stresses from a training session in general or training in particular.

The foot drills are good in the warmup as would be skipping, ankle flicks or some activity that is done one to two minutes or for a total of 50-100 meters broken up into several small reps. The selection and variety here is almost limitless but if the workout is designed to truly train something this portion of the workout can be used to fine tune that training. As a general conditioner were one to do 100m or 200m of barefoot running on a soft surface—I'd have no objection. That is not what happens. One hundred meters soon turns into a lap, then a mile or more, and more is always seen as better.

The main portion of the workout, what most people consider as the workout, would be the development of a theme—aerobic endurance with a long continuous run (45-60+ minutes), anaerobic endurance with two 880s at one's personal best plus 10-15 seconds, lactate tolerance with interval training of repeated 200s or 400s with a set recovery time. This focus will change from day to day and week to week depending on a variety of factors not the least of which are training goals, part of the season, event, age, even sex.

The final portion of the workout is the cool down. What one is trying to do here is normalize the body. From time to time this third phase of a workout can begin with some general endurance conditioning exercises such as circuit training or a limited weight training circuit to work one's overall endurance or general fitness. But even that work will be ended with a cool down period of light jogging, stretching and possibly use of adjunctive therapies such as a flush massage, a short swim or coldwater immersion for 5-10 minutes.

I have heard of athletes doing their barefoot running during this cool down and I would advise against it. The main reason is that at the end of a workout one is fatigued and with fatigue running form or running technique breaks down. Classically technique and skill work are done when the athlete is fresh which is why it is done at the beginning of the workout.

It has often been stated that running is a "ground contact" sport. The forces the feet must sustain with fast running are multiples of 7-10 times one's body weight. The most common training surface for most runners from an industrialized nation is a hard, level surface. The function of shoes becomes twofold—support and protection.

The dominance of the Kenyan nation on worldwide distance running is unparalleled. In the last 40 years the podium placings of Kenyan distance runners at World and Olympic Championships is unequaled. Marathon rankings for the men for 2011 year from *Track and Field News* reveal that 31 of the top 40 marathon times in the world were run by Kenyans. While that level of dominance is unmatched by any other nation in any other event what is truly astounding is that the top 20 times are by 20 different Kenyans!

Kenya is a developing nation suffering from tribal unrest, disease and poor nutrition. The legacy set forth by Kip Keino and Naftali Temu have led to hundreds and hundreds of talented runners on the world stage. Their young athletes often begin the sport from impoverished backgrounds, barefooted and trained on grass and dirt surfaces until adolescence. But interestingly or ironically once the athletes develop the financial means one of their first purchases is a pair of running shoes.

Fashions and fads come and go. Success in sport hinges on one's ability to understand and appreciate what one's training is doing to the body. The opening salt analogy should illustrate the point clearly. Strengthening the foot with foot drills or limited amounts of barefoot/minimalist shoe running can be an important training aid. Trying to design one's training plan around this method is the fast track to the breakdown lane.

Children Running: Can v. Should

The World Records for distance running from the mile to the marathon for 10-year-olds is a graveyard of talent. Those poor guys and girls never do much past that point. Unfortunately, this is a story repeated again and again and again.

Right off—I have strong opinions on this subject. I was a pretty good child runner. I mention this not to brag but to frame my argument. I started running "officially" as a 12-year-old in the New York Road Runners Club back in the days when an event drew 30-40 runners. I remember the unique and famous Fred Lebow being there. He was just unique back then. I was undefeated in the 12 and under ranks. You can look it up if you want.

I always beat the same kid. He was 10 or 11 years old and came up to my hip. Even though I always won he seemed to get all the "atta boy's," it was David v. Goliath and I was Goliath.

I remember talking a number of times with the kid's father. He was a husky guy, maybe 5'9", about 180 pounds and ran in the adult races. He was enthusiastic about his running but never beat anybody. I remember thinking how somebody could know so much and not be so good. I was learning about adults.

I had no coach. The father used to tell me how hard

he trained his son. I distinctly remember one workout he said they did—8x 880 in under 2:40 wearing a 20-pound weight vest. The kid didn't weight 100 pounds. This probably explained his height.

My training seemed to consist of bike rides, some extended walk-jogs and sprint races at practice to see who was fastest. I felt a little guilty winning the races without "really" training.

All I ever heard about was how great this kid was going to be yet week in and week out I beat him like a drum. He had a little brother and I beat him too. Goliath had no mercy.

In high school I ran a 4:30 mile as a 15-year-old and eventually got down to 4:24. Things stalled out there, but I was still running well at ages 30-31. Although the accomplishments never quite caught the hopes, I have much to be thankful for.

When I was coaching I used to get calls 2-3x per year with the voice asking me to coach their son or daughter. The one-sided conversation would go on for five or 10 minutes with the parent rambling on about all the races their kid had won, this 5k, that 10k, town champ, gold medals and on and on. When they stopped to catch their breath, I'd jump in.

"How old is your child?"

"Ten," or eleven or younger.

My advice was always the same. "Buy them a soccer ball, put them in the backyard and call me when they are 15."

There was silence while I gave the parent my two cents. Kids aren't meant to run long distance. Develop their other skills. It is too early to specialize. It wasn't what they wanted to hear. The conversation soon ended, sometimes politely, sometimes with a, "What do you know!"

I know. I was there.

I also know my freshman teams won three league championships in four years. We would have gone four for four but my first year my #3 guy missed the bus the day of the championships. More importantly the teams I left behind by senior year were both the top ranked high school programs in New York State and the Shen team won it all.

Success in the athletic arena hinges on the organization of a "system," talent identification and talent development. It is easy to succeed with the "Box of Rats Method" where all you do is train everybody hard and eventually the top rat emerges. One great rat and a lot of dead rats. The challenge of good coaching is to save the other rats.

Talent identification may be the easiest step. High school recruiting is limited to in-house efforts. I went for numbers. I needed 10 freshmen for cross country. If you had a pulse and could fog a mirror you qualified. I had confidence in my development plan.

The Development Plan—One of the greatest fears of a freshman is—can I do this?

My first words to my freshman teams were, "You will be champions." My practices started the end of doubt. I segregated the frosh and gave them things they could do. We did "destination runs"—run to that tree and back, run to that pole and back, for about two weeks. We rested between runs. We counted heartbeats. I got a clue who had the "engines." After 6-8 of these destination runs, we walked and did push-ups and sit-ups. That was practice until the first race. Oftentimes we ran the first race never having run the full distance. We were usually top five. You can develop from there.

After about two weeks the frosh would start to feel comfortable with it all. They could see they were getting better, a rank order was starting to form and both the quality and quantity of their workload created a momentum on the team that generated enthusiasm. They were developing faith in their abilities—I can do this. A coach can do a lot with a little faith.

This is all well and good you might say but what do you do with a 10-year-old? The best program I have seen is the one championed by the British, the "Five Star Award Scheme." It set the events up with point values and at competitions athletes had to compete in three events. If they hit the predetermined point values, they won a merit badge. The charts were progressive, could be used for various age groups and promoted goal directed behaviors. Incidentally the charts could also be used to identify talent and develop it through an organized system.

Some other points to ponder:

Multilateral development—let kids try many different sports and activities. Up to the age of early specialization, 14 or 15, kids should be exposed to many different physical activities. It helps them in their socialization process, emotional development and problem-solving skills.

Teach fundamentals—I once had a friend who was a great hockey player. He had a friend who as a child was trained as a figure skater, his family would not let him play hockey. As a child he was ridiculed for figure skating. When his parents finally let him play hockey, he became a great hockey player too. He could skate better than anyone on the ice, in fact he could skate circles around them. Movement fundamentals.

The ability of skip is a skill that transfers to many sports and events. Use of baton drills and relays keeps practice fun. Use of hops, skips and jumps makes practice fun. Kids like to do fun stuff.

Train for short distances 400/800m—Short distances prize speed. That is what racing should be about. Shorter races develop tactical sense and decision-making skills in the heat of the battle. Longer endurance runs foster a "grind it out" attitude, obstinance and compulsion—not necessarily the most attractive attributes for a 10-year-old.

Attend events—and not just competitions. Have your youngsters watch the warm-ups and training sessions of better athletes. How does work get done? How do good people act? Carefully pick your role models.

Foster learning—What is the most important thing you learned today? Don't badger the kid with a cross examination but create some introspection. How can they apply that knowledge to the future?

Arrested development—The skeleton of a child is not developed until the late teen years and for some people full growth and development doesn't stop until the early 20s. Excessive exercise or repetitive motion activities can negatively affect the growth of a child. Throwing too many curve balls as a little league pitcher is a prime example. They even have an orthopedic condition called "Little League Elbow."

The very nature of distance running is that of a repetitive motion activity. A thousand steps per mile, mile after mile on a hard surface hitting the ground at 4-7x body weight could potentially damage the growth plates of a child. Nationally they have stopped keeping long distance records for little kids.

There is also the issue of growth. Although I have never seen any studies on this point, intuitively it makes sense to me. If a child trains to excess the energy that the body would use to grow and develop is shunted towards training or competitive efforts. High school rules that allow runners to compete in four events per competition several times a week are short sighted and irresponsible. You can quote me.

Childhood should be a time of exploration and discovery. This includes the introduction to many different activities both social and athletic. Early participation and early success can be both a blessing and a curse.

The entry to high school closely mirrors the recommended age for introduction of serious competitive efforts. A generalized introduction to shorter distance running at that time can begin. At this point the chance of debilitating growth plate injuries are lessened. The comradery of being on a true team offers the chances of participation and decreases the chances of burnout.

A crying, terrified three-year-old with a full diaper makes for a lousy competitor. While the parents might get a laugh at the histrionics I wonder if this develops a psychic association of "new" always being "bad." I can't v. I can.

Once I graduated from the 12 and under class I never heard of the kid in the 20# weight vest again. His road to obscurity was paved with great workouts. The childhood superstars pushed from the start never seem to make it.

Core Stability

Core stability plays a critical role for both the recreational and competitive athlete. While the 6-pack abs may be the obvious result they are more a side attraction of a larger benefit.

Core this. Core that. You can barely turn the page of some health magazine without someone mentioning the importance of the core. There are varied thoughts on core training but past the obvious 6-pack you might be saying to yourself—I think I've seen enough of this.

It is important right off the bat to clarify the distinction between core strength and core stability. Strength is a speed and power quality. Physiology dictates that speed and power is related to the white muscle fibers we have in our muscles. Sprinters, jumpers and throwers, track and field's speed and power events, prize a higher content of white fibers.

Core stability on the other hand is an endurance quality. Were one to do a biopsy of the core muscles one would find red muscle fibers. Core strength is actually a misnomer, our core is not for speed and power as much as it is for endurance, posture and stability.

Posture needs to be viewed in both a literal and figurative sense. Core stability helps with your mother's admonition to "stand up straight" but it also is necessary to position the trunk in such a way that the limbs can be accelerated to produce the running, jumping and throwing actions involved in track and field and most ball sports.

At the corners of the body's core are four ball and socket joints. Ball and socket joints are multi-axial, meaning they can move in every direction. Most shoulders retain this ability throughout one's life. The hip is the body's largest ball and socket joint. Mobility of the hip is significantly less than the shoulder for most people, with the possible exception of hurdlers or ballerinas.

While hip mobility is laudable it can become problematic especially with directed actions. In sprinting the optimal action is straight ahead movement. In fact, any wobbling or side to side type movement at the hip is counterproductive to the sprinter's overall goal of a faster time. But the ball and socket joint of the hip, if not properly stabilized will wobble and exhibit unwanted movement that can decrease one's force production and produce slower times.

The shoulder joint presents with a slightly different scenario. The stability of the shoulder comes into play anytime one tries to push, pull or throw with some force. There are four small muscles ranging in size from about the size of one's thumb to the palm of the hand that initiate shoulder stabilization. Collectively these muscles are called the rotator cuff.

All shoulder problems involve all four of the rotator cuff muscles. No exceptions. And while these are relatively small muscles their injury or dysfunction leads to a domino type dysfunction of the shoulder girdle, across the upper torso to the neck and even problems down the arm to the hand.

The rotator cuff muscles are located on the posterior aspect of the body where they literally remain "out of sight" and out of mind for most people. The muscles are ignored until injured and then they become unforgettable registering pain with virtually every movement of the hand or arm. Rehab of an injured rotator cuff is often slow and frustrating.

While most of one's walking actions are linear most arm and shoulder actions are what could be called "gathering actions." White- and blue-collar workers alike bring their work to their middle or core over and over again. Even the resistance training most athletes go through follows the same pattern. The significance of these gathering actions is that over time they create an imbalance within the rotator cuff. The internal rotation (palm down) rotator cuff muscle, the subscapularis, becomes disproportionally stronger than the two external rotators, the teres minor and infraspinatus.

The next time you are waiting in line take a moment to study the resting position of people's hands. Are they flush against the side of the leg or is the arm twisted with the palm facing backwards? The backward facing palm is a tell-tale sign of a current or developing shoulder problem.

A simple solution to correct this hand pattern is the side-lying dumbbell fly (Fig. 3). This can be done with a can of soup or other weighted object. Start out easy with 10-12 reps and work to 15 before increasing the weight. Perform the grand sweep with the arm first, then place the arm on the flank and perform a smaller sweep.

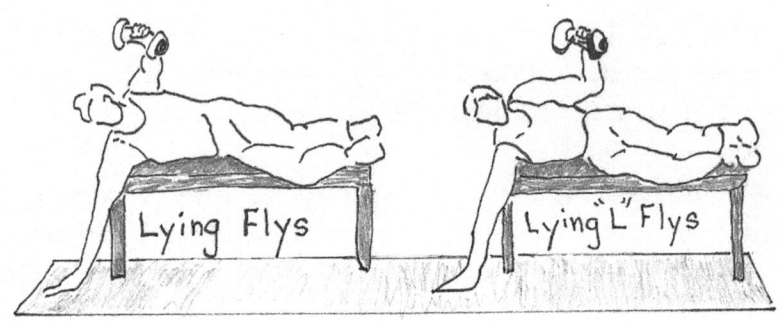

Figure 3. Side lying flys shoulder strengthening exercise for external rotators. Use a large arm sweep for the first exercise (left) and shorter arc with arm resting on trunk (right).

A second option would be to dribble an 8-10# medicine ball against a solid wall or a tree. A little bit of this goes a long way. Remember what we are seeking here is tone of the rotator cuff muscles, not hypertrophy. To create muscular hypertrophy could cause a pinching or impingement syndrome in the shoulders.

The upper core is less of a running problem. Shoulder injuries to runners are rare unless there has been a fall that one has tried to stop with an outstretched hand. Shoulder injuries for the thrower or vaulter are more common due to the use of the arms in those events and a more aggressive weight training program that those events require.

The lower core is a series of muscles that wrap the abdomen top to bottom and side to side. The traditional sit-up may contribute to a beautiful set of 6-pack abs but usually does little to tone the lower core muscles responsible for stabilizing or initiating trunk rotation. (Fig. 4)

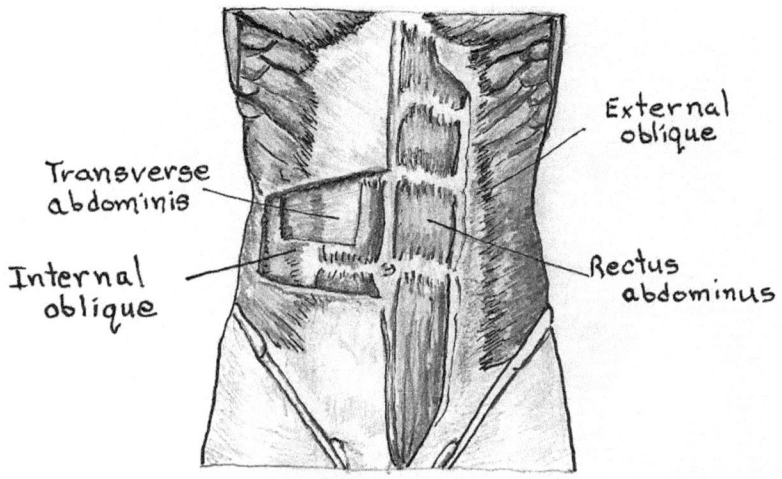

Figure 4. Muscles that wrap the lower core.

One can observe weak abdominal muscles in a runner whose trunk makes it look as if they are wiping down a table. Their arms cross the midline and the shoulders twist back and forth. A complaint weak core runners have when they do speed work is that they just "never feel smooth." What they are noticing is that the shock of ground contact is "jarring" their body. With a weak core there is nothing to attenuate that ground contact force. The solution in part to lower core stability issues is a series of plank positions.

A plank position is basically a push-up position without the push-up (Fig. 5a). It is an isometric contraction of the abdominal muscles. Isometric contractions are those where there is no movement. Isometric training has gone in and out of favor over the last 30 years. Isometrics are actually a highly effective means to make stronger muscle-tendon-bone, ligamentous and fascial plane connections throughout the body. This is an example of "invisible training" of the body that is not seen and generally ignored.

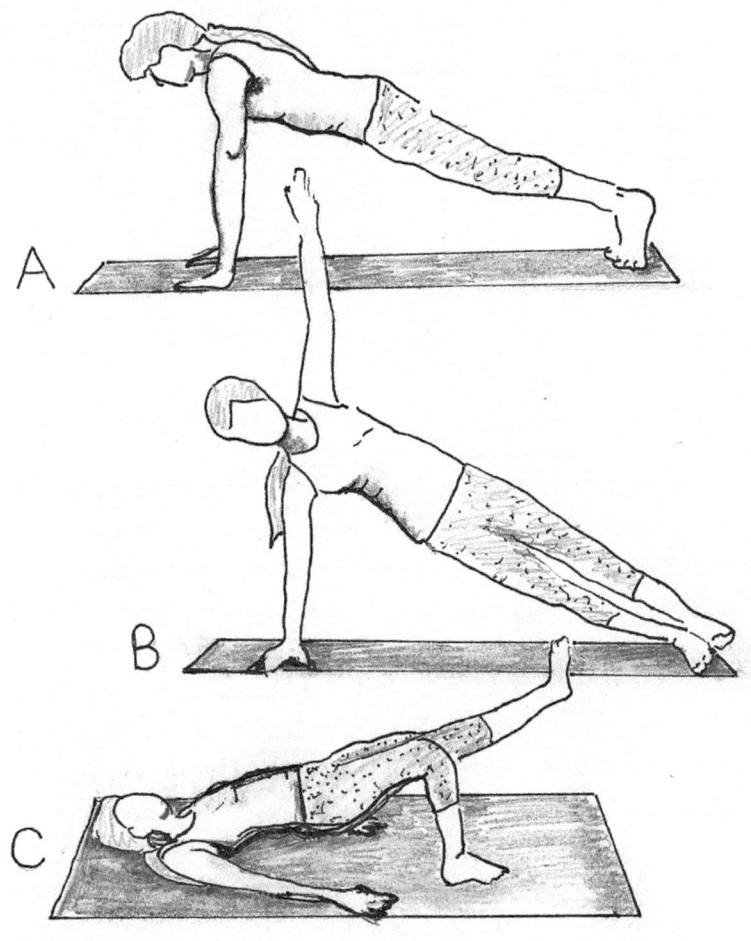

Figure 5a, 5b, 5c. Planks can be held for 10 seconds to start and progress to 30 seconds. With back plank lift hips upward, keep non-ground contact leg's knee straight. Experts question the value past 30 seconds.

Side planks are important to insure all around core development (Fig. 5b). Side stars can be a challenging position that isolates the side of the trunk muscles. A second variation is to lie on one's side and perform the classic yoga move called Side Raise. One can raise the top side leg or lift both legs together to include some toning of the inner thigh. These side planks isolate the lateral aspect of the core. Start out conservatively holding the position for about 10 seconds. Over a week or two increase to 2-3 sets of 10-15 seconds each.

Isolation and stabilization of the back muscles can be done with a back triangle or "dead bug" exercise (Fig. 5c). Keep one foot firmly planted on the ground, raise the opposite leg and maintain a motionless abdomen with the free leg held straight. Once again 10 seconds on each side, alternating sides 2-3 times will tone this area.

Up to this point the traditional sit-up has avoided discussion. While sit-ups were no doubt the staple of most high school gym classes sit-ups have fallen out of favor more recently. There are several reasons for this with the leading one being the stress sit-ups impose on the lower back.

Ten sit-ups do not pose a problem. It is the repeated trunk flexion of 100s and 100s of sit-ups done over time that places excessive wear and tear on the lumbar spine's discs. This area is a problem site for long-term runners (read that as 10+ years or a masters runner). Remember 2/3 of one's bodyweight is above the navel and with each running stride there is a pounding the L5-S1 disc takes as weight is shifted leg to leg. Factor in jumping exercises, high mileage days, an aggressive race schedule, lots of running on concrete surfaces and the occasional stumble and one can begin to see why low back pain is an "occupational hazard" for the serious runner.

Much of the pageantry of thoroughbred racing centers around "the look." Owners buy horses by how they "look." The parade to the post allows the common to see up close what their horse looks like. Even the big hats of Derby Day connect some of the dots of the grand mosaic. But if "the look" was all there was to horse racing every horse would be a champion, every hat worn by a princess and all the railbirds rich. It's not the case.

Over the last 20 years there have been several fitness programs that have championed the importance of the core. While the nuances of each program might slightly differ in total their intent and means to an end help stabilize the body's core.

Core stability is like one's personal values. Values are what one does and how one acts when no one else is watching. With core training the results are not immediately obvious. But it is the long-term benefits that one receives—more productive workouts, a greater work capacity, healthier and more efficient movement patterns that translate to a more productive career.

It is critical that one ask and forthrightly answer the questions—what do I want from all this running? And what am I willing to do to get it? If the core stability concept is new to you, regardless of your level of participation or athletic history, slowly introduce the changes to your routine over the course of one to two weeks. Core training pays big benefits for a small investment of time, usually less than 3-4 minutes of daily practice time. What do you want from all this running? What are you willing to do to get it?

Destination Runs

Can you remember your first day ever of practice? How about the second day? Chances are they were not pleasant memories. The doubt of "Can I do this?" followed 24 hours later by the soreness of newfound muscles leaves one to wonder how you ever made it to the third day of practice. The use of "destination runs," a simple training method to gradually introduce the concept of distance running may simplify this whole process.

Freihofer's *Run For Women* has long had a program where they conduct clinics for elementary schools in the days leading up to the annual race. As a community service national and world class runners take time to interact with local kids introducing the how's and why's of running.

The sessions routinely end with questions from the crowd. Questions are usually simple and straightforward about pets, favorite colors and foods. Recently one of the runners returned laughing how she was embarrassed to be at a loss for words after she was asked, "When you are running, if you know you are going to lose—how come you don't stop running?"

Obviously, the kid didn't get the point. I can say that as an adult with 40+ years involvement in the sport. But what if I am missing the point? Although we do run to win, the results are often different. There is always the possibility of a personal best but that is often not the case either, especially with age. When you give the kid's question a moment's thought—that's a really good question.

The fact of the matter is racing would take on a whole new dynamic if people were stopping as soon as winning hopes were dashed. There would be the occasional sprint to the finish for the leaders but after that the ranks would be thin and the fundraising aspect of the sport would be lost.

The transition of child to adolescent presents a dichotomy of growth and development v. training and competition. Ideally childhood should be a time of discovery. Life should be spent doing a little of this and a little of that. And mostly the "this and that" is accomplished with games.

I use games in the general sense. Read it as unstructured play. The best goal is that there should be no goal. Winning and losing are of negligible importance. When you get tired you stop. The important thing is to have fun and to move.

Concepts like persistence, dedication, drive and always giving your best effort are not on the radar screen of a child. Competition and the need to win do not play such a central role either. Simply put, they are kids. They think like kids and should be allowed to act like them.

But a problem arises when the child has to transition to a more organized setting. The journey of 1000 miles begins with a single step. Organized training has to start somewhere. The challenge is to transition the child into the adolescent athlete in such a manner that the fun of the games can morph into the fundamentals of the sport that will serve one for a career and lifetime.

But think for a moment, that first day of practice must be terrifying for most newbies. No doubt there has been talk of five-mile runs, hill work and the like and all the newbie knows is that they want to stop after one lap of the track.

There is an obvious ability gap here that needs to be bridged quickly or the newbie will soon be on to other things. And these doubts and fears only escalate after one day of practice when the next morning dawns with legs so sore it is difficult to walk.

The point of running is to get to the finish. Conceptually for an adult they can manage the uncertainty of the mid-race void with the faith and confidence that comes from training and experience. The newbie is quickly lost in the void of breathless uncertainty of an unseen finish line.

So the question arises—how does one get the newbie through the void?

What I have successfully used is what I call a destination run. From the first day of practice, after the initial warm-up, we run destination runs. The distances vary from 200m up to about one-half mile.

I would gather the group, point out a landmark (a tree, bench, backstop, etc.) in the distance and give the command to run to the landmark and back. Things were not timed. Speed was at the pace the runner was comfortable with. No walking was allowed.

The newbies returned. I'd have them find the carotid pulse on the neck and count six seconds. Mentally I would start to record exertion and recovery rates. We would walk for a few minutes until everyone "caught their breath." I'd do another carotid pulse check making sure everyone was under 12 beats (120 beats per minute) and send them off to a different destination. This cycle was repeated 6-8 times.

Most will see that this is simply a less structured form of interval training. And doubtless they will be quick to add that this is an unconventional way to do interval training, especially on the first day of a season.

I'll grant the unconventional sentiment but what are the other options here? Most of the runners have never trained. I suggest that any form of distance runs would be counter productive. Even a "short" three miles is a long eternity for a newbie that is too difficult, exhausting and destroys any shred of confidence the athlete may have arrived with. So I would counter with—what is the point?

At least with a destination run there is an accomplished goal that is repeated throughout the practice. With regards to practice the athlete establishes an inventory of successful efforts. They have faced a challenge ("run to that telephone pole and back") and succeeded. Granted, it is a small goal, insignificant when compared with the work of a marathon but it is a brick that forms a base from which greater building can come. A feeling of "I can do this" is the thought of a winner.

Two other points bear mentioning. The rest interval between the destination runs is critical for coaching purposes. No doubt my athletes would remember this as a time for "stories" if at all. But this is where I repeated stories that were lessons on technique, how to act at a meet, what to eat, what to think before a race or how successful varsity runners struggled as freshmen and the personal doubts they mastered allowing them to go on to greater things. The list of topics was planned and presented in 2-3 minutes, a fair rest interval.

And then the first race comes. After the obligatory 15

days of practice, team uniforms and pictures freshmen are ready for the first competitive effort. In the 15 practices of destination runs they may have run some 75+ intervals with nothing longer than an 800 (sometimes we did do a mile time trial).

Inevitably the frosh captain would approach with a team concern about the fact that most had never run the full race distance, usually 1.5 miles. I'd allow him to verbalize this momentary crisis in faith and send him on his way with two quick thoughts. Firstly, I would remind him that the team had completed every workout I had asked them to do in the last two weeks—why would I ask them to race today if they were not prepared to do it? Secondly, I would tell him not to stop until the finish.

Growth and development is an evolution with a little of this and a little of that. The transition of the child to adolescent athlete can be organized in such a way to provide the direction, fundamentals and motivation necessary to create the dedication, drive and desire that will evolve into successful competitive efforts.

Detraining

Recovery happens, except for those that it doesn't. In American we prize ourselves on our ability to make ourselves tired. We spend little time and effort on prescribing recovery efforts that lessen the damage of performance training and may boost subsequent performance. There is a training maxim that says—recover as hard as you train. For many it is easier said than done.

Michael Phelps returned to the US after winning a record eight gold medals at the Beijing Olympics to travel the whirlwind tour of American celebrity. At one point an interviewer asked him what he had done physically during the last 35 days since the Olympics. He laughingly dismissed the question with a simple, "Nothing."

That reply literally turned my stomach. I remember thinking "if that is true, that's not good" for him—or me. In America we do a great job of getting tired. Whether it is the road running community, the three-season high school runner or the madness of the Crossfit disciple the motivation and drive to train is relentless.

The shoe and apparel companies have slogans to fuel this fire that serve as mantras for those days when motivation is low and one's greatest struggle is just to take that first step. We get sold on the idea that the only other life option is obesity and general sloth. Both equally unappealing choices to a motivated individual, even to the point of turning one's stomach.

Consistent training is a series of weeks and months where the athlete cycles through times of stress, rest and adaptation. Some athletes have the intuitive sense to monitor this process on their own, when to press and when to coast. Most need the watchful eye of a coach to provide the carrot or the stick to move things forward. The problem is, the mistaken belief is that one's performance improvement is a never ending spiral upwards. A master's athlete would chuckle at that naïve sentiment. They have already crested the peak of the lifetime PR and have begun to evaluate all life's many facets in an effort to maintain a few seconds here and there.

The other issue many 20-something runners fail to acknowledge is the seasonal nature of sport. For a ball sport person there are set time periods. The pros have a pre-season, main season, post-season and off-season. There are goals for each season. The more responsible athletes do what needs to be done to capitalize on the goals for each season.

For a runner this is a particular challenge. Whether we are talking locally or nationally the opportunity to race year round is there. There was a time when Bill Schrader had a summer road race in Albany's Washington Park and seven people showed up. Odd right? What was odd was this was the only road race in the Capital District for the summer! No Colonie, no Freihofer's, no Boilermaker. Today on any given weekend there are four or more races within a 50-mile radius of Albany allowing the opportunity to race back to back days.

The blurring of the seasons for a runner presents a

challenge as there is always a "next" race. Why this is a challenge is because the body never gets a chance to rest. The body never gets a chance to recover. There is no off season. Those who have done any gardening get this, you have to take some time and let the ground come back.

But for some athletes, Olympic athletes and Olympic team-sport athletes where weather dictates their seasons (think skiing, hockey, skating) these athletes cannot, do not compete in all-seasons. If…

The "if" is the answer to the question—is there a yearly or seasonal plan? Take the swimmer for example (or pick the skier if you like). They train and train to prepare for a terminal championship. Their training raises the ability of the body to adapt to a higher and higher level to the stresses placed upon it. These stresses have been a combination of physical (the muscular strains of training), mental (the continual, relentless drive to achieve one's goals) and the biochemical (the physiological adaptations the body has made to buffer the acidic pH state created by the relentless quest to achieve goals and win). For most of us, if not all, if we were subjected to this triad of stress it would be overwhelming. The results would be physical breakdown, emotional withdrawal or collapse and physical illness. The stress of this level of athletic life would be too great.

But what if you were trained to handle this stress and do it successfully and then go to the Olympics, compete in 17 races over a span of nine days and win eight gold medals and then suddenly do nothing? Nothing for 35 days. Can you see how raising the adaptive levels to such an elevated state and then removing that stress input, that level of physical, mental and biochemical assault to the body that it is suddenly no longer trying to adapt to, that the body is no longer trying to fight, it can present an overwhelming insult and trauma to the body? There is no easy slope for return to normal, there is the drop-off of a cliff.

And in fact Michael Phelps went through significant personal and emotional problems following the Beijing Olympics as chronicled in the November 16, 2015 issue of *Sports Illustrated*. There was a plan to get there (the Olympics) but there was no plan to get *from* there. One can only speculate if this was a failure of his support staff to recognize this or the non-compliance of an athlete expecting to handle fame on his own terms or the impossible demands of American celebrity or a combination of all three.

What resulted was a hyped up system with no place to go. The result for Phelps was a state of restlessness, anxiety, depression, sleep and eating disorders, emotional problems and an inability to cope with the mundane challenges of day to day life. Phelps's return to normal was more an unraveling than a normalization.

That is what detraining is. Detraining is a plan to get from peak condition back to normal. It is a plan to renormalize the body, the mental processes and the biochemical processes. No one is a light switch. While one may have the ability to turn on and turn off effort at will the adaptations that need to take place in the body take weeks and months and possibly years to create. That is training, the "getting tired" bit, remember we Americans do a good job of getting "tired." But if the buildup takes time, so does the ramp down if all this is to be done healthfully.

So what is the average Jane of Joe to do? Train with intention. Most runners seasonally build to a peak over a period of three to four months then take a month "off" to normalize. Active rest, alternate exercise, cross training roughly describes the intent—a movement oriented physical activity that allows for a level of work, while at the same time reducing, gradually easing the stress of performance based training and essentially "allowing the ground to come back."

Part of "The Talk" I always gave my best runners was that they could no longer think like "the led." They could not think like the pack, they had to think "ahead of the pack." Their ability to produce "effort" was their gift. It was made clear that collectively their directed efforts were to be towards times of effort **and** times of rest and regeneration. When this was done correctly the adaptations of the body and the reserves of physical, mental and biochemical energies could be drawn upon, as the effort required. If we could "train with intention," that was how we would win.

Dynamic Stability

Forward motion is more complicated than just putting one foot ahead of another. Dynamic stability is a concept many are either unaware of or disregard but nonetheless plays a critical role in improved performance.

Dynamic stability (DS) is a contradiction of terms. DS can be defined as the ability to hold a posture while moving. There is the contradiction. Posture is a static quality (no movement) while dynamic implies change and movement. In spite of the contradiction DS is a critical component of running technique and the presence or absence of this quality has a direct affect on physical performance and injury incidence.

With regards to running DS can be seen as the ability of the athlete to "post." Posting is biomechanical jargon for being able to rigidly stand on one leg with no side to side sway or wiggle. To the naked eye this sideways translation may be minimal if apparent at all and therefore may be mistakenly discounted as unimportant. But in performance-based sport any deviation from the forward application of force will lead to an increased foot contact time, dissipated ground force and contribute to injuries whether it be the catastrophic failure of a torn hamstring or the cumulative micro-trauma of a tendonitis somewhere in the leg.

There are several muscles that contribute to this concept of dynamic stability in running. It is important to note they all stabilize the hip joint. Remember that the hip joint is a "ball and socket" joint. Ball and socket joints allow for rotary or circular actions. But running is a forward action. The multi-axial nature of the joint allows for the unwanted lateral sway mentioned above. The challenge becomes for one to eliminate the lateral sway while at the same time allowing the complimentary muscles to drive the body forward.

The three main dynamic stabilizers of the hip are the iliopsoas, the glut medius and the adductor magnus. (Fig. 6) When their isometric contractions are coordinated the desired posting is the result. If there is a weakness lateral sway is produced. In fact there is an orthopedic sign called the Trendelenburg Sign that is indicative of glut medius compromise. (Fig. 7)

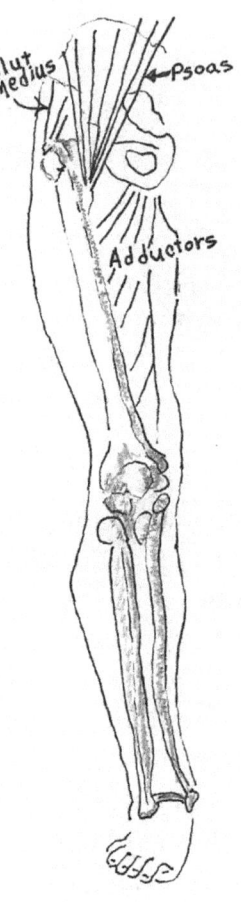

Figure 6. The hip is a "ball and socket" joint. The iliopsoas, adductor magnus and glut medius dynamically stabilize the hip. Weakness or dysfunction here may be evidenced with the complaint of chronically "tight" hamstrings.

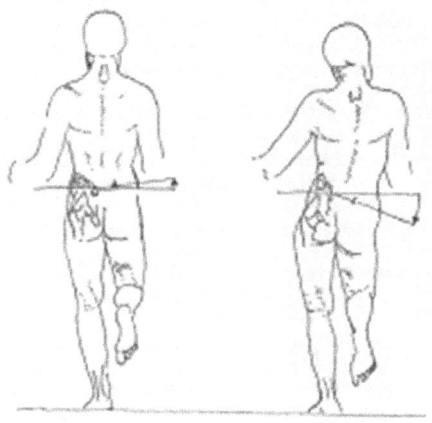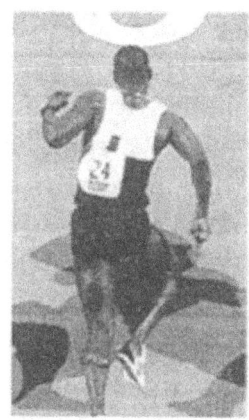

Figure 7. A weak or dysfunctional glut medius can lead to a lateral shifting of the hips or the orthopedic sign called the Trendelenburg Sign. This creates excessive "wear and tear" for a regular human and loss of force application for an elite athlete.

It should be noted that the posterior tibialis also plays an important role in dynamic stability in the foreleg. The PT was profiled in a previous column (*Pace Setter*, December 2011). One of the functions of the PT is to control the velocity of mid-foot pronation. What that means is how fast the foot moves from heel strike to mid stance. The PT controls the three components of how pronation happens. A dysfunctional PT allows for either too much pronation, pronation too soon in the gait cycle or the process of pronation happening too fast. PT can be toned doing the six foot drills on a daily basis and supported by a simple orthotic.

As you no doubt see dynamic stability becomes a cooperative struggle between balance and strength. While one quality may be developed independent of the other when developed synergistically one quality enhances the other.

Why is DS a problem in the first place? Running is a linear activity. For the most part, from the sprinter to the long distance runner what is prized for both athletes is the ability to run in a straight line. Agility or side to side movements come into the mix when one talks about football, soccer or basketball but I would still note that forward or linear actions predominate. After all, the ball fields are longer than they are wide and scoring is achieved by going the length of the field, not the width.

A second reason is that the hip dynamic stabilizers are relatively hidden in the body, effectively invisible. Attention to and development of the dynamic stabilizers does not necessarily lead to muscular hypertrophy. In our narcissistic culture it becomes a situation of "out of sight, out of mind".

A third reason is that without development of the dynamic stabilizers the job of dynamic stabilization is left to muscles that are poorly designed for the job. The hamstrings are designed to drive the thigh backwards and make a minimal contribution towards dynamic stability of the hip. But when forced to provide stabilization of the hip the hamstring twinge, hamstring strain or excessive hamstring "tightness" can be the result. In fact a passive hamstring stretch past 100° of hip flexion that induces hamstring "tightness" is a telltale sign of poorly functioning dynamic stabilizers.

DS becomes a problem because it is rarely a focus of training. As stated above, running is a linear activity. It may also be due to a misunderstanding of the training concept of specificity. Specificity of training dictates that if the primary demand on a system is aerobic, the primary training modality should be aerobic. If the sport is power based then primarily speed and strength should be trained. Running is primarily linear therefore most train the linear quality to the exclusion of other movements. What happens is there is a confusion between "primary and only" with the development of one quality done to the exclusion of the other.

Armed with this knowledge the solutions to the problem becomes relatively simple. One thing that is underscored here is the importance of a solid training plan. That would include not only the long-range planning but also what gets done during a daily workout.

Training the dynamic stabilizers should be done on a daily basis in the warm-up section of each day's practice. This is the portion of the daily practice that could last from 15-30 minutes. If properly designed many of the small, but important details of athletic performance can be addressed. I have often heard runners lament that they cannot budget this amout of time when they only have the lunchhour to do their workout. I have always contended that the time spent here, on the pre-hab/dynamic warm-up is of equal or greater import than what gets done in what most think of the as the traditional workout.

While the ilio-psoas can be addressed with leg lifts and the traditional sit-ups attention to the adductors and the gluts may require some creativity and extra effort. Holding the plank position (Fig. 8a) for 30-60 seconds or doing the plank with hips circles to the right and left will address all three dynamic stabilizers of the hip. Start slowly with three to five circles and build to 10.

Side stars (also called a side plank) will also address all three muscles, especially the glut medius. This is a difficult position to hold and beginning recommendations would be 15-30 seconds on both the right and left sides. (Fig. 8b)

Once the main part of the workout is completed it

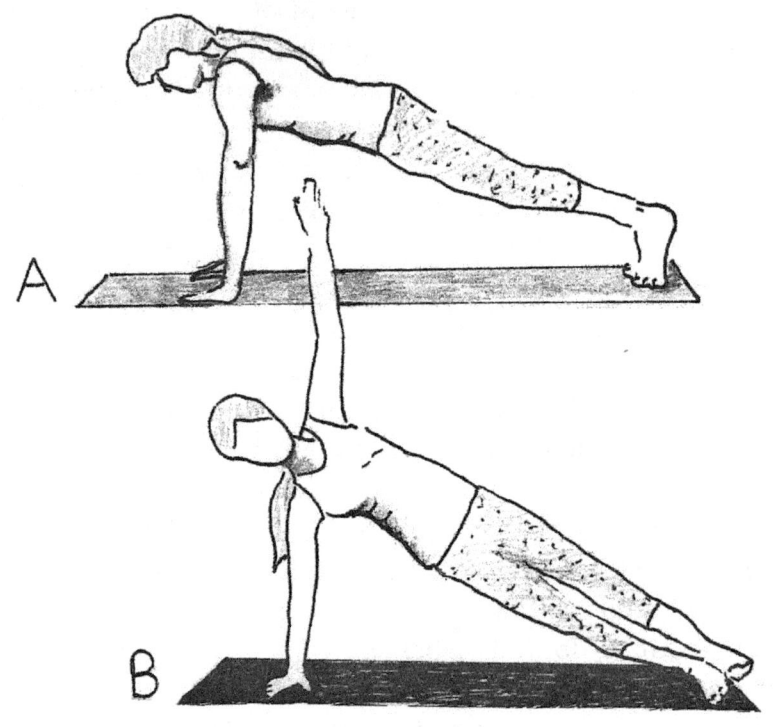

Figure 8a, 8b. Planks can be held 10 seconds to start and work towards 30 seconds.

is recommended to address these muscles with some specific weight training at least twice per week. Traditional squat exercises will help coordinate the stabilizing effect of the muscles but will not specifically address the muscles. While most personal trainers would dispute that statement I refer you back to Figure 7. The sprinter is Ben Johnson who could squat over 500# and still evidenced the Trendelenburg Sign and the posting weakness.

Side leg raises and inward adductor leg sweeps on a total hip machine will isolate and tone those muscles.

While this machine work violates the "train movements, not muscles" rule it needs to be mentioned that we are specifically re-habbing or pre-habbing these muscle groups for the stresses of running and represents an exception to the rule.

In running the flexion and extension of the hip is the fastest volitional movement in the body. This action can be enhanced when the ground support phase of running action is that of a solid post. The development of the dynamic stabilizers in this area will not happen by accident but rather through specific design and intelligent application within a comprehensive training plan. The benefits of such a plan would include improved ground reaction times, a decrease in hamstring injuries ultimately resulting in improved speed actions, forward velocity and performance.

Fun—Commitment—Performance

Children do not arrive with an instruction manual or set of blueprints for their development. Nevertheless, allowing the child to gradually move through these three phases of development will naturally limit the stresses and naturally allow for growth and development.

About 15 months ago I initiated a Skills and Drills program in the Niagara Association that was detailed in the February 2009 *Pace Setter*. While the program has been used only sparingly where it has been used has met with great success.

The Skills and Drills Program is a 6-week introductory course that teaches the entry-level skills of track and field. At a most basic level the athlete learns how to refine the schoolyard skills of running, jumping and throwing.

Since publication of that article I have continued on the exploration of child development particularly with regards to athletics. I teach a course called Elite Sport Science that is a 12-15-hour investigation of modern training theory and all its various facets (work capacity, periodization, biomotor skill development, overtraining, etc.). Within the 20+ topics covered is one on childhood development.

It should be clear to most the demands of elite sport participation and childhood sports are totally at odds with each other. This point is clearly stated in the opening minutes of that lecture. But what is duly noted is that if the child is not "developed" properly there will be no long-term chance of success. The sentiment is neatly summed up with the statement—all things only grow once. The debate over the "right way" rages on.

Childhood development moves through stages. The pure novice is literally a diamond in the rough. They don't know what they don't know, and they could care less. The appeal of sport for many children is to participate in an activity with their friends and have some fun.

In the 90s social researcher Stephen Danish conducted an extensive study of over 3,000 young athletes on the why's and how's of their sports participation. What he found was that the reason some 75% of child athletes quit sport by high school is that the activities ceased being fun.

The experienced, performance minded adult, knows that not all sports participation is fun. Having to do a difficult tempo run or interval training in the cold or rain or when tired is not fun.

What Danish found out was that what most children defined as fun was the balance struck between mastery and challenge. Where there was a balance between mastery (I can do this) and challenge (what is this?) the sense of achievement became a great, enjoyable motivator, something that encouraged participation because it was in a word, fun.

When there was an imbalance between mastery and challenge problems arose. If the task/skill was too complex it generated levels of anxiety (can I do this?) and self-doubt. Conversely if the task was too easy, too simple there was little challenge and the task became boring (why are we doing this?). The art of coaching lies in the ability to strike a creative balance between challenge and mastery.

One of the challenges of athletics is that things do not remain fun forever. With maturity there is a gradual transition from the introductory stage to a stage of commitment. Commitment is a stage where there is a refinement of skill.

Once a series of skills has been introduced and mastered, as physical maturity allows a transition begins to take place. Efforts and energies are now shifted and increased mastery of fundamental movement patterns and skills become more important. Concomitant with this is the introduction of competition that can serve to highlight both one's accomplishments and areas for further attention.

This is not to say that the commitment stage cannot have its fun. Initially there will be the introduction of goals and certain behaviors that are consistent with being on a team. This may in turn require a greater degree of dedication, perseverance, responsibility, teamwork, etc. Clearly this would include the values that one can develop from sport however that is defined. Achievement and mastery of these behaviors elevates one's self-esteem increasing the sense of self-worth, which can be enjoyable, if not fun.

The final stage is performance. This is where the young athlete specializes in one area of sport—as a sprinter, thrower, jumper or endurance athlete. Development is slower. Goals are achieved more slowly but with maturity comes a degree of patience that allows one to forestall the need for immediate gratification.

You'll note that the stages of development—fun, commitment and performance come without defined ages attached. This is by design. Were I pressed to supply ages I'd say the fun stage runs roughly from ages 7-12. The commitment stage runs through high school (13-18) and performance stage begins at around age 18 and continues to career end.

Admittedly these are large windows of time. By right, within each window of time there are further stages of development that could be delineated and benchmarked. This would allow the coach or trainer to manipulate the challenge and mastery variables so that with further skill development there is the motivation to continue.

The limiting factor in athletic development is not enough time. In his book *Outliers*, Malcolm Gladwell notes that the timeline for the transition from novice to an elite mastery of a skill is 10 years with some 10,000 hours of training. In fact, this is an old European coaching adage that is worth exploring for a minute.

Sport does not produce an overnight sensation. Granted gifted individuals like a Tiger Woods or Lebron James may appear to make it look easy but their skills are the result of countless solitary hours spent honing their craft.

The problem for many youth coaches and a significant number of parents is that they act and coach with the assurance that their prodigy is the heir apparent to the current superstar. Frequently, the coach or parent has neither the time, energy, interest, knowledge or revenues to direct a novice to an elite level. Years ago the Canadian Olympic Committee figured out that it took upwards of $2.5 million dollars and 12 years of coaching to get someone to the Olympic 100m finals.

Ten years and 10,000 hours translates to three hours of training a day, six days a week for 52 weeks a year. Anyone faithfully maintaining that level of commitment misses out on a countless number of beers and family barbecues.

Another difficulty with the 10-year window is exactly when does the clock start? If the "go!" begins early in the "fun stage" there is more than a good chance the demands of the sport will outweigh any rewards and participation will cease. Conversely if you begin too late, around age 18, there is a good chance you'll never catch up.

The age of specialization is different for different sports, but it seems a safe guestimation to note that the clock begins to tick as the child enters the commitment stage. Ideally by this time the fundamentals should be set and greater goals become the next step.

It is my hope that adult administrators keep in mind that all things would happen in their time. Highly regimented entry-level programs seem to be a recipe for disaster. For most sporting activities the entry into middle school and high school offers plenty of time for an athlete to develop to their potential. If there is a managed, programmed plan for development the opportunity for a much more fruitful experience in sport is greatly increased.

Hard Level Floors

One of the characteristics of Industrialized Nations is the fact that these societies exist with hard level floors. These hard level floors present a continuous assault on the foot and lower extremity. Improved foot postures and coordination can help alleviate some of these stresses.

One of the things that distinguishes a first order nation like the United States or Canada from the third world or developing nations is the reality of industrialization. Industrialization could be variously defined as an economic superstructure that includes commerce, finance and manufacturing.

One of the requirements of industrialization is the development of an infrastructure that supports and holds together the industry, commerce and finance. The infrastructure involves networks for communication, transportation and distribution of the products. There are also lifestyles associated with this economic model.

But on a very basic level one of the things that differentiates first order and developing nations is the proliferation of cement and hard level floors. At first blush this may seem like an absurd statement, but think for a moment. In your daily life today how much of your time has been spent on a hard level surface? How different would your answer be if you were alive in the non-industrial US of 200 or 300 years ago? Or the developing nations of today?

The more rural your lifestyle (read that as less industrialized) the greater the percentage of time you'd spend on non-cemented surfaces. Consider for a second someone from New York City—there is a real possibility those individuals could go weeks and even months on hard level surfaces, never standing on natural earth. Even the signs in the pocket parks say—"Keep off the grass!"

Were one alive 150 or 200 years ago the situation would be reversed. Most would have done agrarian work where our days would have been spent trudging behind plows over rough fields struggling to scratch out a living. Our houses might have rough cut timbers for flooring but probably not anything approaching the level flooring used today.

So what is the point? With industrialization came the hard level flooring. In part this was due to the mechanization and the assembly line. Both aspects of manufacturing required smooth, unyielding surfaces for the longevity of the machines. Any machine on a cock-eyed floor would wear out faster. Repairs are expensive in terms of down time of the assembly line and lost work.

But what about the "human machine?" Actually, the study of biomechanics was controversial prior to the 1920s because it was thought that comparing or training the human body to act and react like a machine was dehumanizing. Human beings were seen as an extension of the machine and for many jobs simply another interchangeable part. That social dilemma seems rather tame when compared to today's science fiction implications of genetic engineering or stem cell research.

A corollary to my Hard Level Floors Theory is the Weak Foot Theory. With industrialization and the proliferation of cement in our society shoes have become a necessity to protect the feet from the hard, unyielding surfaces. But the shoe wear that has evolved has essentially become a "soft cast" on the foot.

The shoe as a soft cast becomes significant in that the smaller, intrinsic muscles of the foot either never develop properly or atrophy which compromises the effectiveness of the muscles of the foot. This leads to problems in force production by the muscles of the foot and foreleg. Weak muscles cannot maintain proper foot postures and body balance which can create a poor biomechanical foundation for the body. In turn this unstable foundation can create compensation patterns elsewhere in the body or wear and tear injuries like plantar fasciitis or Achilles tendon problems.

All this does not take into account the usually detrimental role fashion plays with footwear. This is particularly true with women's footwear. In the developing world one is fortunate to own a pair of shoes. In industrialized nations not only are the choices relatively limitless but one's choices may also define one's personal taste, occupation or societal status. In our society bare feet are socially unacceptable. If you saw a shoeless child running down the local mall one would almost logically suspect parental neglect.

While the realities of industrialization don't look like they will change in the near future and the visceral appeal of relocating to a deserted island to live off the land may be impractical the truth of the situation is that cement is here to stay.

But there are things one can do to counteract the

stresses posed on the body by modern society that are simple, inexpensive and effective.

Running is a ground contact sport. Because of this it becomes important to prepare the foot for the stresses that athletic participation entails. Listed below are seven simple strategies that if consistently applied should safely prepare the foot for the stresses presented by life in an industrial world.

1. Do the foot drills—When I spoke at the High Performance Summit in Las Vegas in 2005 on improving distance running in America my opening comment was that it has taken me 18 years to get a national audience. I have been banging this pot for a long time. The first five foot drills are done bare-footed and are to: walk on the inside/outside of the feet, walk with the toes pointed in and out, and walk backwards on the toes. The sixth foot drill is to walk on the heels with the shoes on (to protect the heels from bruising). Collectively these drills will tone and strengthen the intrinsic muscles of the foot. They should be done daily for about 25 meters for each drill.

2. Improve your balance—Fully one-half the running action is spent in single support. As you fatigue your balance gets worse. Doubt this? Run a quarter mile as fast as you can and then try to stand still on one leg. Poor balance in the latter stages of training or a race leads to poor foot and leg postures, poorer force production and greater stress and strain on the supporting ligaments and tendons of the lower extremity. One way to improve balance is with a wobble board or balance board. One's balance will also improve dramatically spending one minute a day standing on one leg and then one minute on the other leg. This can be done with the shoes on or off.

3. **Wear quality shoes**—I am not a big proponent of barefoot running. While I have no doubts it will strengthen the foot, barefoot running for most people presents too much stress on the foot and foreleg. A second concern is that of finding an area where one can safely run can be problematic. That being said shoes become a necessity. All the large shoe companies produce quality products. Most specialty shoe stores have many qualified personnel to help with your choice and proper fit. Remember, shoes don't last forever so budget on two or three pair per year.

4. **Try to train on soft surfaces**—Grass and wood chip trails would be ideal and the more training done on these surfaces the better. If that presents a problem local parks with a soccer or baseball field can provide a great jogging surface for an easy recovery day.

5. **Consider an orthotic**—There was a time when I questioned the value of orthotics. Hard level floors are a 24/7 reality in most of our lives. This presents a relentless assault on the foot and the muscles, ligaments and tendons of the feet and low back. As our muscles fatigue they promote poor foot postures. An orthotic, which admittedly is a crutch of sorts, helps support the arches of the feet and reduce the stress on the joints and soft tissue above the foot. Podiatrists, pedorthists and chiropractors have the training to design a functional orthotic. Even a generic, off the shelf orthotic can offer some support and relief.

6. **Lift some weights**—When I give advice regarding running I try to focus on things most everyone can do with the least amount of equipment. Strengthening the quads is an exception. If you do not belong to a gym you'll need to purchase a leg extension machine and some free weights. Most sporting goods stores carry a simple leg extension machine for less than $200. Consider it a

lifetime investment. The leg extension exercises create a strong quad and a great shock absorber. If you strengthen the quad you stabilize the knee. Two sets of 15 reps done twice weekly will strengthen the quad greatly for the stresses of running.

A second exercise addresses the hip stabilizers. Tie a piece of rope at your shoulder height and duck your head back and forth under the rope. This swaying bob and weave is an old boxer's exercise that works the muscles of the inner and outer thighs which help stabilize the leg when one is standing in single support. Over the course of two weeks work up to 100 reps.

7. Sit like a yogi—Sitting cross legged like a person who practices yoga will give a good stretch to the lateral ankle which allows the foot greater dorsiflexion. Why is that important? When you run there will be less strain on the gastroc-Achilles complex as you toe-off and less likelihood of a calf pull or Achilles strain.

The reality of hard level floors will probably not change in one's immediate future but a proactive mindset can prepare the foot, legs and body for the stresses athletic participation and running are likely to present to the body. Detailed above are some simple solutions that may add 30 minutes of training time per week but will enhance one's ability to train harder, longer or faster all with greater safety.

Havana Dreaming

I proposed going to Cuba to interview Alberto Juantorena and got the okay from Track and Field News. *Supposedly it was okay for educators and journalists to travel there. This was in 2005. I made the trip. I'm glad I did. Someday things will change. The country was beautiful, but very much frozen in time, for better or worse.*

I went to Cuba.

Now before you start running at the mind with some secret government work or participation in tortuous deeds at Gitmo the truth is I was on assignment for *Track Coach Magazine* to interview Alberto Juantorena, their great Olympic champion.

Q.—Alberto, what is your role in sport now?

The trip down was pretty painless. At Cuban customs there was a bit of a snag. I showed my credentials and explained the reason for my visit. I mentioned Juantorena, to which the official asked, "Juantorena?" And three quick thumps of his stamper later I was on my way. But then the officer called me back and with broken English said, "How about Marion Jones?" She had just gotten her jail sentence that week. Luggage in hand, all I could do was shrug.

On the bus ride to the hotel our tour guide was a red-haired spitting image of a guy I coached in college. I'll call him "Red." The guide was a tourism student from the University of Havana. His English was okay, a little drawn out in places where he searched for a suitable word or phrase. But to warm-up the crowd Red told jokes, American jokes.

I had never heard an American joke before. I marveled at this. The bus was mostly Canadians and Red got more than a few chuckles. I just sat there, nice and quiet and thought to myself—welcome to the world.

Red—What sound does a Cuban toilet make when flushed? A.- George Bushhhhh…

For a fleeting second, I entertained betting Red that I could sing the Cuban National Anthem. You probably know it too—"Row, Row, Row Your Boat…," but in the interest of international relations and self-preservation I shared that private moment with myself.

Q. Alberto, your career began as a basketball player. How far did you go with basketball?

The first time I saw Alberto Juantorena was at the Montreal Olympics. He was speeding down the backstretch of the 800m semis. He immediately stood out. He was reputed to have a 10' stride but even at 9' his stride length greatly contrasted with the rest of the world. I noted this over striding to my friend and that "this joker will never last." But he did last which may explain why he was running on the track and I was watching from the cheap seats.

Q. Alberto, did you really have a 10' or 3-meter stride?

Juantorena went on to run seven races in seven days and won the golds in the 400 and 800m, a feat that has not been repeated before or since. He was the dominant force in those events until 1980 when an Achilles injury ended it all. He was the first Cuban track Olympic champion and arguably one of the greatest runners to come out of the Caribbean.

Q. What did winning the two golds mean to your post-Olympic career?

For most people reading this column Cuba is shrouded in mystery and has been that way our whole life. The Cuban Missile Crisis was part of some of our childhoods and we all know now how safe we would have been hiding under those elementary school desks had something really happened.

Since Fidel Castro took over, Cuba has all but fallen off the map. If you watch the national weather reports Cuba never gets mentioned. Especially during hurricane season. It is like they are the 10-ton elephant in the kitchen and nobody wants to see it.

Q. Alberto, how much weight did you lose running seven races in seven days?

One of the things I did not realize about Cuba was its size. Cuba is 700 miles long and 200 miles wide! If you were to take that land mass and lie it over the US it would stretch from Virginia to Maine and cover 60% of the US population. Although my travel in Cuba was limited one of the things that strikes you is that there is nobody there. Cuba has about 11 million people and it seems that they are all in Havana.

While that is not quite true once you get out to the countryside, you are in the country. Where I stayed, Varadero is about 90 miles from Havana. In 90 miles you travel through one city called Matanzas and a lot of nothing. The coastal road is all seashore with an occasional cinderblock house.

My impressions of Cuba ran hot and cold. Having studied in the Soviet Union (in 1983) during the Cold War I got to see the archetypal communist country firsthand. Cuba proved to be different in a number of ways.

Q. There is a perception in America that Cuba and the Soviet Union had a completely harmonious relationship in sport and politics. Is that true?

First of all, they had churches and bookstores and the place was pretty clean. The vast majority of people looked well cared for. They wore functional but not fashionable clothing, everyone seemed well fed and they had good teeth. Cuba has a socialized healthcare program that exports doctors throughout the world. Controversial filmmaker Michael Moore has chronicled this in his documentary *Sicko*, which is worth a watch.

Q. Cuba has been internationally recognized as having an excellent healthcare system in spite of shortages of medicines and technological advances. Why is the Cuban system so successful?

In Havana there were any number of bookstores and the titles were wide ranging from the expected political commentary of Ché Guevara to biographies of JFK and Martin Luther King. The books were expensive, even by American standards and I can't vouch for the contents but at the used booksellers you could get pretty much anything you wanted including original pictures of Fidel Castro during the Revolution.

On the flip side was the country's infrastructure. My impression is that Havana is melting. The old building facades are 50+ years old with most all stained by the soot of time. While there are sporadic renovations taking place that restore the former beauty to the building it only serves to heighten the contrast with its aging neighbor.

Public transportation is weak. There was a bus system in Havana but in the outlying areas we were advised not to use the public transportation as it was regarded as unreliable, slow and overcrowded. There is a railway system out of Havana called the Hershey Railway, after the Hershey Bar family who built it back in the 50s or before.

And there are the cars. Most have seen programs on all the old Cuban cars. They are all over the place. My guestimate is that 40% are vintage Olds or Chevys or some other outdated classic. And some are beautiful. While I am not a car buff by any means I did stop a number of times to marvel as one of those classic beauties drove by. Time in a time warp.

You don't get much on Fidel Castro from anyone. (He was reported ill and had not yet ceded power to his brother.) That was another big change between Russia and Cuba. There are no murals or pictures of him around. I asked one of the bus tour guides why that was and she told me that it was because Castro did not want to create a cult of personality. On the other hand, Ché is everywhere. If you were to combine the Golden Arches, the Wendy's girl and Rachel Ray that would approach the marketing presence of Ché. Books, posters, t-shirts, murals, coffee cups and on and on.

I asked about this too and it is because Ché, as a 20-something, represents the Revolution, the ongoing revolution. I'm sure some buy into that but I'm also sure many wish the Revolution would soon include better jobs, American TV and a Wal-Mart or two.

There is a biography on Fidel Castro by Tad Szulc, the *New York Times* Caribbean correspondent for years, that proved to be an excellent reference for the trip to Cuba. It helped explain many things. One needs to understand some of the larger political and economic concepts like imperialism and how this misuse of American economic interests have shaped the Caribbean, Central and South America. For better or worse Castro has been one man who stood up to those economic interests and lived to tell about it.

Q.—Alberto do you foresee the improvement of Cuban- American relations anytime soon?

I don't expect to see the thawing of Cuban American relations anytime soon. In large part it has to do with the fact that when Castro took over Cuba he nationalized all the businesses and took away everyone's property. This led to the mass exodus of Cubans to South Florida. For the US to recognize Cuba and normalize relations would validate Castro's actions and negate any future claims the expatriots had. There is a lot of land in a 700-mile long island.

Q.—They have taken baseball out of the Olympics—how disappointing has that been for the Cuban people?

As for the interview—I didn't get it. Everything got okayed through the censors in the Office of Propaganda and Public Relations but Juantorena was attending a meeting in another part of the island and was unavailable the day I made it to Havana.

I was very disappointed. I felt I had many good questions that would have allowed Juantorena to explain his and his country's perspective on a number of athletic, political and economic issues. Major cultural shifts can never be reduced to a simple dichotomy and what has always fascinated me about meeting and interviewing people is trying to understand who their intellectual influences were and how their thought processes evolved.

Would I go back? Not as things are now. If there was a normalization of relations and travel became less restrictive I probably would. But when and if that happens there will be an explosion in development and the time-warp images I've seen will become all but a memory.

A Wrinkle in Time

Ed Neiles, Pace Setter editor at the time, called and asked if I had any "special remembrances" for the 25th anniversary edition of the Pace Setter. Before I hung up the phone, I knew what I would write about. The 1982 Christmas Rush had to be it. Special thanks go to Mike MacAdam, Tom Dalton, Miles Irish, Bob Oates, Bill Shrader, Jr., and Jim Gibney.

The Christmas Rush Indoor Track Meet was the largest combined open/high school/college meet in the Capital Region. When I started the meet 14 years ago one of my goals was to create an "everyman's" meet with opportunities for Junior Olympians through Masters. Although the meet was notoriously long it was always a meet for all athletes.

In the early 70s there were no open indoor track and field meets to speak of in the Capital District. If you had the interest and ability you could catch a Trailways to the 168th St. Armory in New York City and spend 18 bucks and 10 hours traveling for a two-minute race. It was tough being famous.

I got the idea for a local indoor meet from Bill Shrader. To say Bill was one of the driving forces behind distance running in the Capital District minimizes his contribution.

In the late 70s Bill would put on a January indoor meet in Albany's Washington Avenue Armory. The floor of the Albany Armory was slick like ice. The fact that Barry Brown ran meet records of 4:10 in the mile and sub-nine in the two mile speak to his remarkable ability.

One of the first things I did when I got hired as the track coach at Union was to plan a large indoor meet. One of my goals was to open up the Union facility as much as possible to the high school Tri-County Indoor Track League and give open runners a chance to run on a good facility without having to travel 3-4 hours to Boston or NYC.

The December meet date got reserved and my bare bones marketing plan called for getting the local AAU/TAC involved. Somebody told me to contact Bill Shrader from the Albany YMCA. I remembered Bill from the Albany YMCA's Summer Jamboree races he put on each July in Washington Park, a meet dubbed "The Shrader Invitational" because it annually showcased his talented children. I got 5th in a five-mile field of nine once—running in the old days.

I called Bill to tell him my plan. He told me of a new group for track called The Athletic Congress and invited me to the next meeting.

At the meeting I made my indoor meet pitch to which George Regan, the new Adirondack TAC president suggested I make this meet the Adirondack Indoor Track Championships. It didn't seem quite appropriate to make a December meet, the first meet of the year a championship, but it would add prestige to the meet. I accepted the offer.

I have one vivid memory of the first Christmas Rush. The equipment cage that stored the cart with all the shots, starting blocks, tape measures, medicine kit, etc. was stuck closed. In my haste to get the meet going on time I pulled the door open with a poor grip. My hand slipped and my thumb caught the wire mesh fence. In no time there was blood everywhere. I got two Band-Aids and wheeled the cart onto the track floor. The show must go on.

At the January TAC meeting I gave my report. The meet ran long but no one got too fired up. George Regan was particularly enthused noting that since I had the "motivation, drive and desire" to put on a large invitational maybe I'd be interested in a position as Chair of the Adirondack Men and Women's Track and Field. I accepted that offer too.

The early TAC meetings were held in the back of the Albany YMCA. Freihofer's was in its infancy but the running boom was happening. Road races were growing and the Albany area boasted many talented runners headed by Barry Brown.

There was a time, as impossible as it seems, when race awards were only given to first, second and third places—period. There were no age groups. Age group racing is one of Bill Shrader's legacies. Bill, as any meet director will attest, was always a champion for the rights of seniors. You'd feel a little tug on your sleeve to find Bill standing by your side with the opening, "You know what you should do?" A question he was poised to answer.

Bill was always very nice to me. Whether or not he saw me as one of the people to carry on his work he never said. I do know that if I ever had a question, he always had time to share his knowledge and wisdom with me.

"You know what you should do?" Bill began. "You should put a 60-and-over 4-Mile Relay in the Christmas Rush."

First, I think he's kidding. If I learned one thing from the first Christmas Rush it was that we were trying to cram 12 hours of meet into eight hours of schedule. It wouldn't fit.

"I could get Dan Geer, Bill Brobston, Jim Gibney to run with me."

But Bill was serious. I listened to him but I'm thinking why not a pregnant ladies 440? That might lead to some excitement.

"We could set the World Record for the 60-and-over 4-Mile Relay...it's soft," and Bill drew that "soft" out before he brought the thought to a close with his little imp smile and the little he-he-he laugh he used whenever he'd made his point and won. I said I'd "think" about it.

There was no way. My dilemma was four old guys running 40 laps around a track, there would certainly be only one team and we'd be lucky if they broke 28 minutes. That figured to be 30 minutes of dead time in a meet already behind schedule.

But the secret to good promotion is to give them something to remember. I fully realized my decision was going to get me hung by the high school coaches. I sat down to write the entry form for the Second Annual Christmas Rush and put the "60-and-over 4-Mile Relay" smack dab in the middle of the high school program.

Once Bill gets the okay, he assembled his team. Bill's team ran under the banner of the Capital Track Club, but they had never met each other. Designated to run was 62-year-old Jim Gibney from Schenectady, 63-year-old Dan Geer from Vermont and 67-year-old Bill Brobston from Saugerties. Bill was pushing a legal 65.

Out of the blue Jim Gibney got a call. "Is this Jim Gibney the runner?" Gibney had only been running three or four years and was thrilled with the designation and invitation.

Gibney told Shrader he figured he could do a 6:30 mile, the same time the other three guys hoped for. The record was 28 minutes and change held by the Syracuse

Chargers. According to Shrader's calculations they figured to break the record by an easy two minutes—the record was "soft." On schedule they showed up, warmed up and were called to the line. Pete McKay was the voice of the Christmas Rush. I always liked to have Pete on the mike. He spoke clearly and articulately. He understood the meet and he knew track. He was there when you needed him and otherwise remained quiet.

"Please clear the track." Pete introduced Geer, Brobston, Gibney and Shrader. He went on to say that they would be attempting to break the World Record for the 60-and-over 4-Mile Relay. Amid puzzled looks and idle chatter the start gun cracked and off went Gibney on his solo journey.

Ten laps later Gibney handed off to Bill Shrader. Gibney ran a 6:15 mile split. Bill carried on and finished his leg in an identical 6:15 split. Brobston, who to this day remains one of the top age-group runners in the world, got the stick.

The best place in Union's Field House to watch a meet was from the announcer's stand. Generally I never got to watch many races. As clerk, assistant starter or referee I was always running from one fire to the next. Midway through Brobston's leg I made it to Pete.

Brobston's half split was a little over three-minutes Shrader's team was a good two minutes up on the record that won't be broken but rather shattered. I see Bill waving at me from the floor. I tell Pete, "Get the track clear, they are going to do it."

"Please keep the track clear..." Pete makes the announcement and everything stops. Here is one old guy chugging along and every high school kid in the place is cheering and clapping and waving him on. Brobston hits another 6:15 mile split and hands off to Geer and 6:19 later, total time 25:04.9, Bill Shrader and the Capital Track Club had a World Record.

I look at Pete and say, "What could top this?" There was a warm buzz about the building. Bill Shrader had done so much for so many. As those four old guys jogged their victory lap a wide-angle lens couldn't have captured their smiles.

A few minutes later I'm back in the thick of the meet. We did have one big event left, the Brooks Invitational 3000m. Barry Brown was scheduled to race. Also on the card was Siena standout Tom Dalton, John Underwood and high schooler Miles Irish.

Dick Stevens, Irish's coach convinced me to let Miles into the invite. Miles had a good fall campaign, but I felt he wasn't ready to get "thrown to the dogs." I signed him in anyway.

John Underwood, from Johnstown, had recently relocated from Eugene, Oregon where he had run an 8:48 steeplechase. Rounding out the field was Tom Dalton. Dalton had been a cross country All-American for Siena and was turning back all challengers as the area's top runner. A month earlier he had beaten Barry Brown in Schenectady's fall classic, the *Gazette Stockade-athon*. On paper we had great race.

As a meet director, the thing I hated about invitationals was that it was like planning your own funeral, the only person sure to be there was you. On paper we did have a great race. Unfortunately, that is usually where the race remains, but then, one by one all four guys showed up.

Pete MacKay did a graceful introduction and starter Bob Oates called the runners to the line. There were some big egos on the track that in many ways represented the past, present and future of running in the Albany area. Underwood jumped to the lead and hit the quarter in 63 and the half in a too fast 2:08. I made my way back to Pete's perch at the announcer's stand to see who would be the first to blow up.

Underwood pushed the pace through a 3:14 1320 and a 4:23 mile. All four guys ran in single file. The announcement of a 4:23 mile split drew gasps. The place was starting to go nuts. "Please clear the track!"

Tom Dalton called this race his "breakthrough." He remembered the race vividly. "It had great interest. The race was right at the end of the high school meet. With Miles and Barry we spanned all age groups."

A month earlier, while on a warm down after the Stockade-athon victory, Miles Irish approached Tom Dalton and prophetically stated he was going to break the national high school records for the 600m, 1000m and 2 mile in the coming winter. "It wasn't like he was bragging, just saying," says Dalton. But with a 4:23 mile split Miles was hanging on for dear life.

"I remember distinct things," began Miles. "We hit 4:23 for the mile and ran the next 440 in 62 seconds. I was over my head." Dear life indeed.

With three laps to go Dalton and Brown pass the slowing but not faltering Underwood. The race for the lead is strength (Dalton) versus speed (Brown). Speed always wins. Barry Brown passes Dalton with two laps to go. I'm not believing my watch. A quick figure has these guys running a low 8-minute 3000m, equivalent to a mid-8:40 two-mile. Dalton chases Brown into the last lap.

The gym is bedlam. Brown leads Dalton into the last lap, but Dalton won't quit. From up above it's looking Brown, Brown, Brown until the final straight and here comes Dalton. Tom charges down the final straight to beat Barry by a step in 8:11.9. Unbelievable! All but forgotten I look up to see Miles run through the line in 8:16. I do a quick conversion and figure Miles broke nine minutes for 2 miles. I'm stunned. I say to Pete, "Miles just broke 9 minutes," and Pete, so caught up in the excitement of the race booms over the PA, "Miles Irish just broke 9 minutes!" Underwood "faded" to 8:19, converting to another sub-nine clocking.

Miles Irish's third place 8:16.1 was the third fastest indoor high school 3000m ever run behind Gerry Lindgren and Jeff Nelson. Nelson later broke Steve Prefontaine's outdoor 2-mile record.

When I called in the meet results to one of the New York City track magazines the question I got from New York was, "Who counted the laps?"

I didn't have an answer. Two weeks later Miles Irish did. In a meet at Lehigh he broke the NYS indoor mile record with a 4:10 mile. Thirty minutes later he ran a 1:52/800m relay split. Later that winter, as predicted, he set national high school records in the 600m and 1000m. Nobody questioned lap counts again.

This past December in Atlanta at the USATF Convention I ran into John Underwood. We had dinner and after a few minutes of general catch-up started talking about the race. I told John he made the race. If he had not pushed the pace no one would have ever run those times. "I ran to win," was his comment. This past summer John won the World Masters Steeplechase in a solid 9:14. He's never lost the fire.

The meet results of that day are checkered with the area's most famous track names. NCAA champion Kevin Scheuer won the mile and 800m. Joe Zelezniak threw 63' in the shot. Albany State coach Roberto Vives won the 50H. Deiter Drake won the 12 and under 800m. Junior National Champ Jim Mann won the walk. Andy Urquhart won the master's mile. OJ Kastberg beat Dom Colose in the open 3000m and Tim Layden, Fred Kitzrow, Kevin St. John and John Shannon won the two-mile relay.

The women's meet produced their own who's who. Monica Osterlin beat Inge Stockman in the mile. Chris Bergeron won the 3000m. Mary Beth Allen beat Laura LaMena in the high school mile and Tom Miller's daughter, Melissa won the 12 and under 800m.

Jim Gibney and Dan Geer still hook-up for an annual age group clash at the Thanksgiving Cardiac Classic. Brobston is still a world force for his age group. Miles Irish went on to star at Georgetown and owns his own business in California. John Underwood has become one of the top experts in the world in the physiology of training and hopes to break Ken Popejoy's American masters mile record this winter of 4:12.9.

Tom Dalton has refused to fade into his late 30s and remains one of the dominant runners in the area, state and Northeast. Bill Shrader and Barry Brown have passed on to greener pastures, although Barry's demise still confuses us all.

In the grand scheme December 11, 1982 was just a wrinkle in time, but for Shrader's Raiders, the four guys in the Brooks Invitational 3000m and the hundreds in attendance it was a day of special moments.

"I ask myself sometimes, was it really me?" says Miles Irish with more than a twinge of wonder. "And then I just feel fortunate to have been part of the whole thing." A sentiment that can be sung in chorus.

Hittleman's Yoga

*By chance an overheard conversation when
I was in a desperate state led to a find that
changed my life and has become a life-long guide. Yoga
touts the development of balance, poise
and grace and gave me back an athletic career
when all my "experts" said it was over.*

One day when I was a junior in college and having a boring day at practice, I decided to give the hurdles a try. One misstep lead to an 18-month ride on the medical merry-go-round that ended my collegiate career, seemingly ended my athletic career all together and certainly changed my life.

I had injured my back and no one knew what to do. There was a rapid succession of ineffective hot packs, expensive "I don't knows" and even one joker who was convinced it was all in my head. This was in spite of the fact that at one point I could hardly walk, couldn't sit or stand for any length of time and for over a month couldn't reach my hands below my knees.

The low point was the day I went food shopping. I loaded up my cart and proceeded to the checkout. The problem was I couldn't get the food out of the cart. Some old lady behind me had to help me get the food on the belt. While I was tremendously grateful, I was at the same time devastated. I was in the prime of a promising athletic career that had been reduced to semi-invalid status. My anger and frustration were crushing. I had to do something.

Therapy suggestions from teammates, coaches, friends and relatives were frequent and varied. I tried just about everything. I even tried yoga. Somewhere in my eclectic book-of-the-month club collection I had a copy of a how-to yoga book. As I paged through it the contents only fueled my futility. Pictured was an emaciated half-naked man with his feet tucked behind his head, bent over backwards with his feet on his head and one where he put a string up his nose and got it to come out his mouth. While there was no doubt some voyeuristic value here attempting any of the postures or procedures in my current condition was probably dangerous and out of the question.

The one thing I could do, albeit on a limited level, was lift weights. At that time the college's weight facility was archaic but there were enough dumbbells and rudimentary machines that I could do something. Often, I would see one of the college's professors doing stretching—it looked like stretching to me, anyway. I overhead him tell a colleague that he had traveled overseas and gotten hepatitis and couldn't exert himself until it cleared up. "So," he said, "I just do yoga every day."

What he did didn't look like any yoga I had seen in that book. There must be another book. There was. What I found at a local bookstore was Richard Hittleman's *28 Day Guide to Yoga*. As I scanned through the book I noted several immediate changes. First and foremost the stretches or what he called postures were pretty simple. Secondly, they were progressive in nature. It was a guided self-study. There was a plan and the title stated it—it took 28 days. The paperback cost $1.95 and that changed my life.

In truth I could not do all the postures. I still was handicapped with limited range of motion and almost constant pain. But as I progressed through the book I began to notice I always felt better after a lesson. And a weird thing I noticed was that I slept better. It took a while to recognize this but ultimately an evening session lead to a subsequent morning when I felt like I had an extra hour's sleep.

In the initial days I would do simple postures that as the body loosened up, in time, became slightly more challenging. At the end of each day's lesson was a short motivational thought that tied in the day's moves, explained how or why this form of yoga worked or explained the why's of certain changes that would be occurring—like better sleep.

Although my collegiate career was lost, I was able to recover from my injury to the point that within three years I was training and racing pretty much as I chose. Certainly, any success I had in my late 20s and early 30s was directly attributable to an almost daily practice of Hittleman's Yoga.

Yoga can be variously translated to mean control, join or unite. The various forms of yoga strive to develop different spiritual qualities. Hatha yoga's goal is to purify the body and probably is the first step or a steppingstone to other yogic disciplines. Raja yoga involves meditation on the higher spiritual ideals of self-control, blissful awareness and positive love. Karmic yoga is the practice of a union of thought and action. An example of this practice would be selfless service to humanity—like how Mother Theresa has been portrayed. Another example would be the "random acts of kindness" extolled by the bumper sticker but practiced on a continual basis.

Hittleman's Yoga is predominantly a brand of hatha yoga. While there are other types of yoga that seem to come in and out of vogue, I have always stayed with the hatha yoga and Hittleman's simple but effective plan. Hatha yoga is a form of yoga that as a discipline prizes posture, graceful movements, diet, breathing and meditation. Taken together attention to these actions helps refresh and rejuvenate the body. If such forces as gravity and aging conspire to "knock the blocks down" a routine of Hatha yoga will go a long way towards restacking the blocks on a daily basis.

As mentioned above, Hittleman's book is a self-study guide and is progressive in nature. I have recommended this book to countless patients and athletes. In fact, the small bookstore where I live started to carry five or six copies all the time because I sent so many people to get a copy as part of their rehab plan. When I coached we always had a copy of the book on the equipment cart along with the jump ropes, medicine balls and balance boards. If an athlete was injured or had something like mono they would come to practice, do the yoga and still feel a part of the team.

In all the clinics I have done Hittleman's Yoga book is always on my short list of recommended reads just for that reason. I literally have recommended the book a thousand times.

Interestingly there are some secondary benefits I got from the book that made me a better teacher and coach. I began to see and over time allowed the book's methods to develop in me an intuitive sense for progressive development and how an intellect or one's athletic skills can unfold with nurturing, and the patient turn of a calendar page.

Oddly when I studied in the Soviet Union and asked one of my professors if the Russians did yoga they were dismissive on the subject. To coach in Russia one had to have been an athlete of sorts and produced a master's level thesis on some aspect of the event or sport one was to coach.

The Russians had in fact studied yoga but found it to be "non-competitive" and something that did not contribute to this focal aspect of sport. I was stunned and this bothered me for a long time until I realized that this was very much consistent with their coaching philosophy where every day was "very much hard work." They spent little time on rest and recovery. And then I checked the stats—who can name a world-class Russian distance runner in the last 25 years? And if you could how long did they stay at the top? The Russians, sans yoga, have only had flashes of success and much quick burnout.

Although one would be hard pressed to find a copy of Hittleman's Yoga for $1.95 the current price of $10 is an investment that will pay dividends long into one's athletic career and life.

If one follows the directions in the book I feel safe recommending Hittleman's Yoga to almost anyone. It will prove to be a great education on how the body responds to progressive challenges over time. There are motivational and informational tips and clues that add to the development of the total athlete or total person. For the competitive athlete a 20-minute daily routine will provide enough "margin of error" so that one can safely train a little harder or a little more due to the increased flexibility, improved suppleness of one's joint capsules and the overall function of the various systems of the body. Finally, for those on the mend Hittleman's Yoga offers a safe alternative to a medical merry-go-round that is often not so merry and frequently a journey to nowhere.

Hyponatremia

Water intoxication seems like a ridiculous problem. But it can happen and does happen even with the vigilant athlete who closely monitors their hydration schedule. The state of one's skin (wet, dry or grainy) post competition can give clues that can be life-saving.

One of the limiting factors of athletic performance is the elevation of the body's core temperature. While a normal body temperature of 98.6° F may be present during times of rest prolonged exercise may increase the core temperature to 106°F/41°C or in some cases higher. The body uses its water and its fluid stores to dissipate this heat but with perspiration these fluids must be replaced, hence the age old recommendation "to drink."

An ambient temperature of 55°F/13°C seems to be the point which heat can affect athletic performance. It is interesting to note that over the decades countless world and national records have been produced in the cooler, late summer evenings of Scandinavia.

In the old days of running "to drink (water) or not drink" was a very real question. To put this in perspective I am talking about a time before the running boom, Gatorade and Runner's World.

Any knowledge of the subject was more of the locker

room variety passed along by aging sages who were just as likely to know what they were talking about as not.

Hydration, particularly during and post workout or competition, followed various schools of thought. It would cause cramping. It had to be at room temperature. And it better be clear. You need to remember at one time soda and sugared "juices" were the only fluids other than water readily available. Distilled water was sold in grocery stores but that was for your mother's electric iron. To buy water for consumption was a ridiculous idea. Adding to the problem was the fact that there were no screw caps for the water jugs.

But as the study of physiology advanced with tread mill runners as the main subjects such things as perspiration rates, core temperatures and the perils of dehydration crept into the consciousness of the running community. The benefits of water were rediscovered and this "new" understanding was championed far and wide.

As the 80s and 90s wore on the social status of completing a marathon became a mark of accomplishment for many runners. Everyone was doing it. Actors and actresses, the formerly sedentary on a personal crusade, even mammoth pro football players switched venues and pounded out the 26 miles.

All the while water, clear water was touted as the magic solution for the physiologic stresses of longer endurance. But then some astute finish line EMT's and physicians began to notice something odd. Race finishers were beginning to present with a series of symptoms that were not those of classic dehydration. Oddly, the ailing runners had been drinking water, plenty of water before, during and after the competition yet something was obviously wrong.

In fact, the well-hydrated athletes were suffering from water intoxication, they were drunk on water. No doubt the first time one hears this there is a high level of incredulity. How can this be? There is no natural alcohol in water, but it all has to do with balance. The intoxication has to do with fluid level imbalances.

When we talk of balance here it is not of the postural kind but rather chemical balance. The body strives to maintain its chemical balance, a part of homeostasis, in a number of ways.

Everyone knows that exercise raises the core temperature of the body and the body sweats to cool itself off. This is the body's attempt to approximate homeostasis and on an elementary level led to the recommendation to replenish the lost sweat by drinking water. Simple and sensible.

But what one needs to remember is that sweat is not just "water" but rather a complex mixture of minerals, salts (taste your sweat) and body wastes in a watery solution. These minerals and salts are the components of the electrolytes referred to on television by the energy replacement drinks such as Gatorade or PowerAde.

If we return to the balance concept for a moment, one needs to accept the fact that there is an ideal ratio of water to sodium to potassium and other minerals. Now consider for a moment the stresses any longer endurance event has on the body. If significant percentages of water and sodium and potassium and other minerals are sweated out during exercise and only water is replaced it should be obvious that in the subsequent state homeostasis has been significantly disrupted. There is too much water and not enough salts (particularly sodium, low sodium = hyponatremia) the results of which are hyponatremia and water intoxication.

It seems logical that this all cannot be that serious, after all it is only water. Unfortunately this statement is false.

Depending on the amount of the water intake signs and symptoms can range from an upset stomach to nausea, headache, confusion, hallucinations, seizures, cerebral edema and even death. There is an infamous hazing incident at NY's Plattsburgh State where fraternity pledges were force fed quarts and quarts of water and one of the pledges died.

So while the importance of water during strenuous exercise cannot be discounted it becomes equally important for one to consider the inclusion of electrolyte replacement drinks.

But the question remains, when is water drinking enough? Numerous factors can significantly affect one's perspiration rate including fitness level, heat and humidity over the preceding days, previous food and fluid intake, over the counter and prescription medications, time of the event, sleep patterns, clothing, wind and cloud cover.

Considering the effects of all these conditions make it obvious that high level athletic performance is not just showing up to an event 15-minutes early and having your shoes double-knotted.

For almost a decade I have directed the chiropractic services for the Rochester Marathon. It is a race day that includes a 10K, half-marathon and a full marathon. All races start together and the runners finish with an escalating problem set dependent on their time of activity. As the full marathoners straggle in their presentation is very telling in terms of recommended re-hydration strategies.

All the marathoners finish with an elevated core temperature. As a rule it is important to cool the body down whether it be with wet towels, immersion in a water bath or by a simple bottle shower (water poured over the head). Experience has taught that marathoners fall into three general categories following a race.

If the marathoner's skin is wet and they are still sweating they are usually well hydrated. General recommendations would be to continue with the cool down, stretching, re-hydration and a light snack.

If the marathoner's skin is dry this could be either the early or late signs of heat injury. It is better to err on the side of caution. Use of the above stated cooling methods, re-hydration with both water and electrolyte replacement drinks are recommended and close monitoring for 30-60 minutes is warranted.

The potential hyponatrimic athlete presents with "crusty skin." These dried salt stains usually form on the jaw, around the armpits and forearms. The uniform may also have a starched feel to it from the dried salt. The grainy feel is the telltale sign that the athlete has lost significant amounts of salt electrolytes, particularly sodium. For these athletes the recommendation is usually drinking 100% electrolyte replacement drinks.

Ironically there have been cases of hyponatremia that have occurred due to drug testing. At the higher levels of sport athletes are routinely urine tested for performance enhancing drugs. The problem for some athletes is that following a hard effort on a hot day the last urge of an athlete may have is to urinate. Regardless of their "desire" athletes are sequestered and given all the water and time needed to produce a urine sample. There have been cases where the athlete has become over hydrated and developed hyponatremia as a result of trying to produce the required urine sample.

Competitive efforts create a situation where multiple

factors need to be considered for one to safely and successfully compete. Re-hydration along with a sensible diet is the bedrock of a safe and quicker recovery. As the mysteries of the body's physiology continue to unfold awareness of such advances allows one to train more efficiently and compete more effectively with the real possibility of safer superlative efforts.

Incidental Exercise

Lasse Viren, the four-time Olympic distance champion was reputed to walk up to 12 miles a day in addition to his training. It probably had little effect on his cardio-vascular endurance, but it was a significant amount of time spent on his feet. This article was originally published before the time of cell phone apps that can now conveniently record one's daily steps.

Sooner or later one's running and exercising goals start to change. The training goal of 30, 40 or 50 miles a week becomes less realistic due to injuries, family commitments or the aging process. But for those who have caught "the bug" and lifelong fitness is "the way" a beckoning sedentary life can be problematic.

The task then becomes choosing a suitable pursuit that will safely offer the benefits of fitness within the confines of a busy schedule and without the risk of debilitating injury.

One common denominator in most everyone's life is walking. Walking is our primary means of ambulating, but it also can be a great exercise. Authorities vary in their walking recommendations from daily to alternate days. But the reality is that to some degree we walk everyday—can't that count for something?

In fact, it can. By chance I caught a short report on National Public Radio about how the Japanese are monitoring fitness, insuring they get enough exercise on a daily basis to maintain fitness. My ears perked up, because if there is a culture that has made compulsive behavior a fine art it is the Japanese.

What many Japanese have done is start wearing a belt pedometer that counts how many steps are taken daily. Every time the center of gravity is raised about two inches the meter clicks. The goal is 10,000 clicks or steps per day. They figure that 10,000 steps is what is necessary to burn off the energy of a 2200 calorie diet and provide a constant challenge to the cardio-vascular system that will maintain a level of fitness.

Upon close inspection there are several things that are beautiful about this system. The pedometer measures steps, not distance. This is a good idea because it eliminates all the debate about tall and short people, longer and shorter strides, who weighs more or other concerns that cloud the issue. The bottom line is the same for all—10,000 steps.

Another nice thing is that the meter is potentially always on. Suddenly you come to realize that a bad parking slot is not the tragedy it once was. In fact, you might pick something at the end of the lot because it allows you to get in another few hundred steps. Stairs versus elevators also become more appealing. And if you have to mow your lawn you might chose the push mower over the rider... well, maybe not, but you see the point.

Mathematically consuming a 2200 calorie diet means burning up about one calorie every five steps. I'm not sure how that jibes with the meter on the StairMaster but the NPR report contended that consistently hitting the 10,000 number will not only maintain cardio-vascular fitness but also maintain weight.

For those interested in losing weight the formula becomes to simply up the daily steps to 10,500 or 11,000 while maintaining the same caloric intake and through time the pounds will melt away. Researchers in the Arizona State Physiology Department have been doing studies in this area with promising results.

To get started you need a pedometer that registers steps (not distance). Walk4life.com on the Internet sells several models that run about $25.

To begin your program I suggest charting your daily walks for two weeks to a month. You will be surprised that 10,000 steps is a "long day" and probably will make you more tired than you would think. I suggest slowly building to the 10,000 steps. It is also interesting to try to guess your daily steps by judging your evening fatigue. With practice you'll be able to predict your number of steps by how tired you are.

For those who need to know 10,000 steps works out to roughly six miles worth of incidental exercise. But as stated above I think you'll be pleasantly surprised that 10,000 steps presents for a relatively fatiguing day, and that day-in, day-out consistently hitting 10,000 steps will be a challenge.

Fitness should be a lifelong goal. The fitness of a day begins with a single step. With the aid of a pedometer measuring daily steps one can rest assured one had gotten some daily exercise even though it might not come through the more traditional means of putting on the shoes and banging out the miles.

Linear People

As we age our movements become more linear in nature. While children play "tag, you're it" all the time, this is not an activity engaged in by the elderly. The repercussions of this linear movement can have a significant effect on one's immediate performance and long-term health.

One of the odd things about life, that we never seem to think of, is that as we age we become more linear. What I mean by that is that we tend to travel in straighter lines. The significance of this is that there are implications for our body that affects our health, well being and athletic performance in both the general and specific sense.

There is an old adage that applies here—use it or lose it. Whether it be knowledge, skills or physical abilities what gets used gets sharpened, that not used gets lost. That is how the musician or athlete develops a talent and the couch potato loses theirs.

The particular problem this causes for an adult, and for this discussion "adult" refers to anyone past the teen years, is becoming more linear leads to the atrophy of the medial and lateral stabilizer muscles of the body.

The 20-something (or 30-something) is not a child anymore, at least not physically, and subsequently does not engage in the activities of a child. Specifically, I'm talking about the running, jumping and games of childhood. Of course, there are exceptions, athletes who may continue to play sports like basketball or soccer well into middle age but I would counter that even those individuals would benefit from attention to development of their medial and lateral movement skills.

Now it would make simple sense that medial and lateral development would be part of the competitive athlete's training plan—but more often than not, it is not.

And for the competitive runner it becomes worse. The nature of sport dictates and prizes one's ability to move quickly in a linear manner. Lateral movement represents time lost through dissipated force production and an increase in the time one's foot is on the ground—the ground reaction time. Two critical concepts we'll come back to.

What is lacking in many training regimes, no matter what the sport, is attention to the concept of multi-lateral development (MLD). MLD can be partially understood by discussing the concept of physical fitness. Physical fitness is classically defined as the ability to meet present and future physical challenges with success. If one considers that statement for a moment it becomes obvious that the application of the concept would vary greatly from athlete to elderly person. And it would also vary significantly from sport to sport.

MLD ideally should be a training component in the early part of one's training calendar. If a training calendar is divided into four larger areas of training focused attention to MLD should have a strong emphasis in the early general development phase, early in the training cycle. Attention to MLD is decreased, but not abandoned throughout the training calendar and is the underpinning link between general and specific training.

So what should be addressed with MLD? If we take a second to define what is means to be an athlete that will give some greater direction. An athlete is a subtle combination of balance, poise and grace coupled with the physical speed and power necessary to successfully compete. Accepting this, how does one develop these skills?

Training can be done in a joint by joint approach (bodybuilding) or by training specific movements that address multiple joints at once, or at least in sequence. While there is validity in both approaches the vast majority of sports involve the broader physical concept of movements. But it is also critical to give attention to specific joint complexes, such as the hips, that may present as a "weak link" in a kinetic chain. This weak link can become a focal point of injury or a lack of development that translates into unrealized potential through dissipated force production or an increase in ground reaction times.

A second area for consideration when constructing a training plan is for one to design workouts that involve the whole body in an exercise. Use of Olympic lifts (snatch or clean and jerk), squatting and various other exercises using body weight or free weights can challenge several combinations of muscle groups at once. This is a good idea because if the exercises are chosen carefully one can structure the workout that would mimic the demands of the competitive activity.

Another movement-type area is attention to core stability. The core can be safely defined as the area from the shoulders to the groin, generally referred to as the trunk. Any balance work on the large physio-balls will help create core stability. How this works is that the small, intrinsic muscles of the spine, the oblique muscles of the lower torso and the stomach muscles must work in unison to stabilize the hips, pelvis and lumbar spine before any activity can begin. A stable core is truly the basis of any power and speed activity and should be an initial area of concern.

A third area for consideration are dynamic movements that again challenge the body in multiple planes of motion. Sideways running, cross-over steps, side lunges or more esoteric actions like t'ai chi, Somatics or yoga all can challenge the dynamic stabilizers of the body reducing any lateral sway or counter productive movements that dissipate forces reducing biomechanical efficiency.

The last point, but certainly not the least is that functional development of the dynamic stabilizers will go a long way towards injury prevention. Maximal use is always abuse. It becomes important for long-term health and well being of the athlete that any training regime be designed to include work to lessen this damage, what some have called "pre-hab." Attention to the development of the dynamic stabilizers is just that.

Balance must be struck between the general and specific nature of training. They both play a significant role for the recreational athlete and the performance-based athlete. The awareness and realization of the subtle demands of sports performance often becomes one of the factors that differentiates one from achieving the benefits of an active lifestyle versus the frustration and limitations of nuisance pains and injury. So while the shortest distance between to points will remain a straight line the fact is that the most productive path will include a few zigzags.

Overtraining

One of the great difficulties of being self-coached is that there is no one around to pull back on the reins. Blinded by one's own personal interests the athlete self-motivates him or herself into an injury or illness. The body will give some tips when it has had enough. If only we'd listen to them. And if the time comes when good enough is never enough, get some help.

One of the things most athletes pride themselves on is the ability to "go the extra mile." That cliché translates to different things for different sports. It may be one more drill, another set in the weight room, another interval or literally one more mile. From a psychological standpoint this mindset of "one more" can translate into the mental toughness necessary to push past the point of fatigue, even pain and produce a superlative effort.

We see this all the time. The media champions superhuman feats that both amaze and inspire. But all this extra effort comes with a cost and raises a thorny question. When is enough, enough? Or even more troubling is the associated mindset that "good enough is never enough."

There is a fine line between training and overtraining. Fatigue is a defense mechanism of the body. This reality may be ignored by the novice but it is always on the mind of the competitive athlete as the consequences of overtraining, illness and injury, are a sure brake to athletic development.

Overtraining (OT) may be defined as a physiologic state where the misguided athlete has mistakenly transitioned from work as a productive, strengthening activity to work where one's effort exceeds the body's ability to recover from the stress with illness and injury the long-term result.

The body adapts to the stresses placed upon it—to a point. Modern training is about stress management. If the stress is manageable the body gets stronger, faster or "healthier," however these qualities may be more fully defined. This cycle of stress can be represented by Yokalev's Model (Diagram 2). The three components, stress, rest and adaptation are the three components of all training.

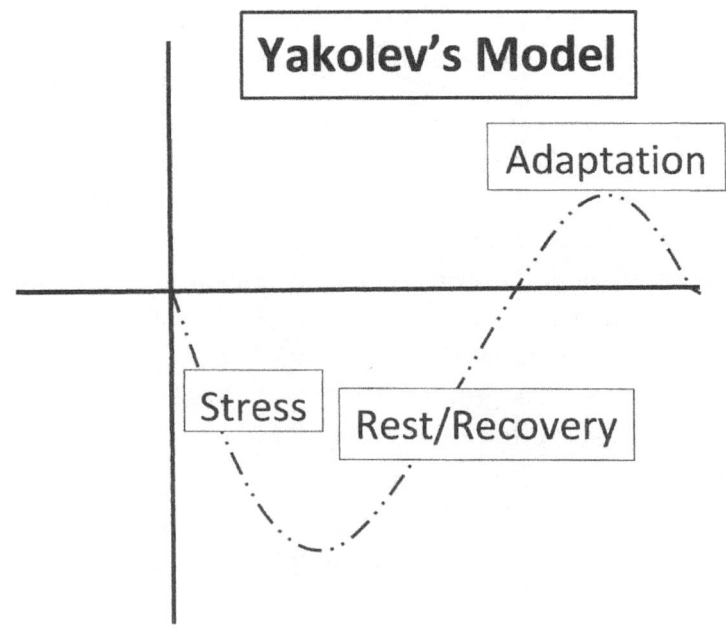

Diagram 2. Yakolev's Model is the adaption of Selye's G.A.S. model to sport. Training is a series of repeated cycles of stress-rest/recovery-adaptation.

The real key to understanding this curve is the role rest and recovery play. One of the catchy maxims that is starting to circulate within the athletic community is that one should "recover as hard as one trains." On the surface that statement may seem like nonsense, as the implied effort of "hard" is the polar opposite of the passive rest.

But what is meant here is that rest should not be a passive process but rather a disciplined, organized activity that allows one to maximize the benefits of nutrition, sleep, and other factors such as flexibility, hydration and mindset. When viewed in this light rest is something that can be actively done "right" or passively done wrong.

OT can become an issue when there is little regard for one's recovery or when the workload exceeds the body's ability to recover. In truth OT is really a fatigue continuum that progresses from fatigue to overreaching, overtraining and finally illness and injury. (Diagram 3) The most telling

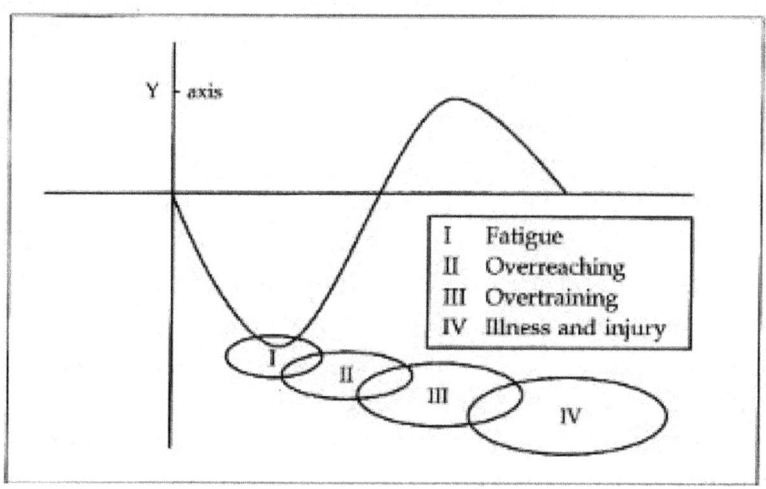

Diagram 3. Yakolev's Model with the progressive nature of
I. Fatigue, II. Overreaching, III. Overtraining and IV. Illness/injury.
Note the possibility of increased lost training time as the severity of overtraining progresses.

factor in all these states is time. Note that the deeper one progresses in the fatigue states the longer one may remain there and the more difficult it is to return to normal.

In recent years the understanding of OT has evolved so that now fatigue syndromes are divided into two pathways—neural and metabolic. Speed and power athletes (sprinters, shot putters, and weightlifters) whose competitions depend on explosive bursts of the sympathetic nervous system are prone to develop neural OT. It is believed this type of OT is due to exhaustion of the axioplasma, the "blood" of a nerve. The combination of lack of recovery, poor diet and poor training design all conspire to produce neural OT.

Metabolic OT is more a general system exhaustion affecting the parasympathetic nervous system. Metabolic OT has a slower onset with depletion of the system happening over time due to long-term imbalances of an acidic body pH, poor nutrition or a chronic lack of sleep. Long distance runners and triathletes are more apt to suffer from metabolic OT. Diet plays a more central role in metabolic OT. A habitual narrow food selection repeated week after week slowly depletes the body of essential nutrients and the energy reserves of the body.

There is a psychological overlay to both types of OT. Both neural and metabolic OT are characterized by a loss of motivation. Coordination, concentration and the ability to relax also suffer. Many of the signs of melancholy or slight depression are similar to that of OT. While depressed individuals may not be athletic by any means nonetheless it is fair to say these individuals may be "overtrained" by life.

One of the points emphasized in the December 2013 *Pace Setter* column on "Training Theory" was the importance of cycling through a series of hard-medium-easy days. For one to expect positive results after a series of hard, soul killing days of work is both unrealistic and dangerous to the body. While all this work may be part of the "plan" I would argue strongly that it is a misguided plan that will eventually lead to physical breakdown.

This raises the question as to how a coach or athlete could monitor stress and fitness levels or can this even be done? In fact, something as simple as monitoring one's morning heart rate will give a good indication as to how one has recovered from the previous day's work.

What needs to be established is a simple baseline of morning heart rates over the days of a season. A consistent number will emerge. If, for example, a series of 60 beat mornings is one's baseline a spike of 10% or six beats per minute is a sign one has not recovered from the stress of the previous day's workout. An easy day with some extra rest is in order.

A second method, equally effective is to test one's morning urine pH to see if the urine is acidic or alkaline. This can be done with a simple strip of litmus paper (MicroEssentials pH range 5.5-8.0 available from most drug stores). Acidic urine signals an alkaline body physiology (this is good). Alkaline urine signals an acidic body physiology (this is bad) which is the result of overtraining, poor diet, not enough rest or a combination of the three indicating that the body has not recovered from the previous day's workout.

Other early telltale signs of OT include a steadily decreasing body weight. This is not the preferred monitoring method as high levels of fitness can dictate losing some weight. A second method is how well one tolerates cold. In a healthy, resilient state momentarily stepping into the cold without a coat is no big deal. When you are physically run down the chill to the body is immediate.

A final telltale sign is loss of motivation to train. When the excitement of practice has become such a grind that simply putting on one's shoes is a chore a few days off or an alternate physical activity are in order. This speaks to the psychological overlay of OT mentioned above.

Just as the wise farmer understands the importance of seasonal crop rotation in maintaining healthy earth the experienced athlete accepts that one cannot healthily train the same way with a high level of intensity day after day.

Fatigue syndromes progress on a continuum. More work is not necessarily better; you cannot beat a dead horse. Smarter work is better. Insecurity causes one to over prepare. While this may have short-term benefits in planning a meeting or a business trip it is frequently disastrous when applied long-term to an athletic career. The "one more," extra mile and 110% effort mentality are all sentiments that will eventually lead to breakdown.

Sacrifice, dedication and hard work will always be the cornerstones of outstanding achievements. The pursuit of excellence can never be a sometime thing. Training with intention is a critical factor but so also is recovering with intention. Directed recovery efforts allow one to optimize the results of hard work and effort. OT in all its gradations is an avoidable state when one applies some knowledge, self-monitoring and simple rest.

Plyometrics

I have been long known as one who discourages the use of plyometrics. The problem is not that they don't work (I think they work very well) but rather most athletes are not adequately prepared for the heightened stresses associated with these exercises. Plyometrics are not a conditioning exercise but rather something that challenges that last little bit of ability from a highly trained athlete.

It seems that with some regularity I catch a magazine cover in a supermarket line extolling the virtues of plyometric exercises. It makes me cringe. Inevitably it is a magazine marketed towards the weekend warrior with life's tips digested down to 3-7 quick, easy steps. Plyometric training does not easily digest into quick, easy steps.

Traditionally plyometrics has been synonymous with "jump training." And while various forms of jump training certainly qualify as a form of plyometrics, it is not the only form. Plyometric training can be done with the arms, abdominal muscles and other muscles of the trunk.

For the highly trained, performance-based athlete plyometrics may prove to be the icing on the cake, that little workout that bumps one up to the next achievement level. For the inexperienced, the marginally trained or someone with a misguided self-assessment plyometrics will almost certainly produce a rapid breakdown or injury.

In the "old" days the LSD crowd (long slow distance advocates) used to chide their interval trained competitors with the adage "speed kills," meaning that fast running leads to breakdown. In fact, there was an ounce of truth to that statement. Indiscriminate use of speed work, without proper preparation and recovery will cause breakdown. But it can be argued that properly applied with adequate warm-up, flexibility and proper dosage speed work can significantly improve one's performance technically and tactically.

Nonetheless used inappropriately by an untrained or poorly trained individual speed does "kill" and following that reasoning, if speed kills, plyometrics will kill faster.

How do plyometrics work? Plyometric exercises, in theory, sharpen the reaction time, which is closely linked to one's ability to apply force. It is one's ability to apply force, over a short period of time that produces power which is an essential element of speed actions.

So if plyometrics are an essential element in speed development why do I have such obvious reservations regarding plyometric use? Bottom line is that athletes are generally NOT physically prepared for the stress plyometrics generate on the body. Force plate studies have been done that indicate there is a momentary stress of 10-20x one's body weight with some jumping exercises. Many people like to quote the adage—if it does not destroy you it makes you stronger. For the poorly conditioned that destruction comes in the form of a rip.

What rips? Generally, it is the connective tissue where muscle transitions to tendon before it attaches to bone. Repeated micro-injury to this area causes a tendinitis—

such as an Achilles' tendon injury or a shin splint. If you have ever suffered a calf pull you can certainly identify.

For the highly trained plyometrics do have their place. There needs to be a substantial amount of preparation work done prior to their use. You can read that as a training history of "years." When doing heavy leg jumps a good gauge to use is if one can squat 1.5x body weight. Another gauge is the ability to triple jump over 40 feet. If squatting with weights or triple jumping are not part of your weekly routine—skip the use of plyometrics.

Secondly there comes the issue of landing—does one use a single or double support method? This means landing on one or two legs. I happened to observe one of Tom Tellez's (coach of Carl Lewis) workouts. He had all of his guys landing double support. I asked him why. His answer was short and to the point—they get hurt more often when they land on one leg, single support. That worked for me.

How many jumps should one do in a practice session? This is called "ground contacts." In Russia they used early season workouts approaching 80-100 ground contacts building towards 200 in a single session. Again, I asked Tellez how many ground contacts his guys did. He told me he never counted. He watched and timed the drills. Once the athlete started getting slower the session ended. Plyometrics should train explosiveness, Tellez told me, not endurance. That worked for me too.

So are there any plyometric drills that everyone can use? Simple things like line hops, skipping, strides or doing strides with a 3-step and jump are all easy leg plyometrics that any trained athlete can use, even children. Box drills (jumping from or to or to and from a 12"-24" box) are better reserved for the mogul skier or highly competitive triple jumper. For those readers I suggest some of the writing of Don Chu. Check the Internet.

Remember that plyometric exercises can also be done for the arms or trunk. Exercises using a medicine ball can be used to develop arm speed or develop strength and coordination. One drill we used consistently was called "talking arms" where one dribbles a medicine ball against a concrete wall. This develops stabilization strength of the rotator cuff muscles (the shoulder stabilizers) but also wrist flexors and grip strength.

I used to do a speed and performance clinic where one segment dealt with plyometric use and many of the cautions noted above. During a break two coaches from a leading women's college basketball program sheepishly approached me and asked what does one do after an athlete had inappropriately used plyometrics. It seems the coaches had attended a "jump higher now" clinic two weeks before and used all the drills and injured five of the 12 women on the team. It is tough getting the Genie back into the bottle.

With plyometrics an honest evaluation of one's ability and performance goals are essential. The importance of preparatory work cannot be ignored. Finally, when using the exercises, when the speed of the action slows, the drill is over. Adherence to these simple rules will allow one to safely use this form of exercises that may add that little extra to boost one to the next level.

Pronation and Supination

Pronation and supination are biomechanical terms that are frequently bantered about in the athletic community. Understanding them on a deeper level helps one design training routines that will strengthen the foot and ultimately enhance performance while at the same time making athletic participation safer.

When writing for a running audience one has a pre-selected group, fitness sophisticated far above the average Joe. No doubt there is at least a basic appreciation for proper nutrition, the necessity of preventive healthcare measures and some scientific understanding of physiology, biomechanics and training theory as it applies to the sport.

Ask any runner about the terms pronation and supination and most would be able to accurately demonstrate either of the two foot positions with a simple "foot turns in (supination)" or "foot turns out (pronation)" demonstration of the concepts.

But if one were to dig a little deeper and ask why pronation is important or why supination is important, well, now we've struck upon "a good question."

At various points in the gait cycle all healthy feet pronate and supinate. It probably could be argued that the human foot does not need to do this but the counterpoint would be that a foot that does not pronate or supinate will affect how one walks and probably preclude any type of running and legally could be seen as a documentable disability.

But what exactly is pronation and supination? As the foot goes through ground contact it acts as either a mobile adapter (pronation) or as a rigid lever (supination). Understanding the concepts of the mobile adapter and the rigid lever are central to explaining why pronation and supination are important and the role and function the human foot plays in running or walking.

We'll examine supination first. When one lifts up or dorsiflexes the great toe the foot becomes supinated. (Fig. 9) This is in part why the coaching cue of "knee up—toe-up" is used to train sprinters. Raising the great toe elevates the arch and "locks" all the small bones of the foot making

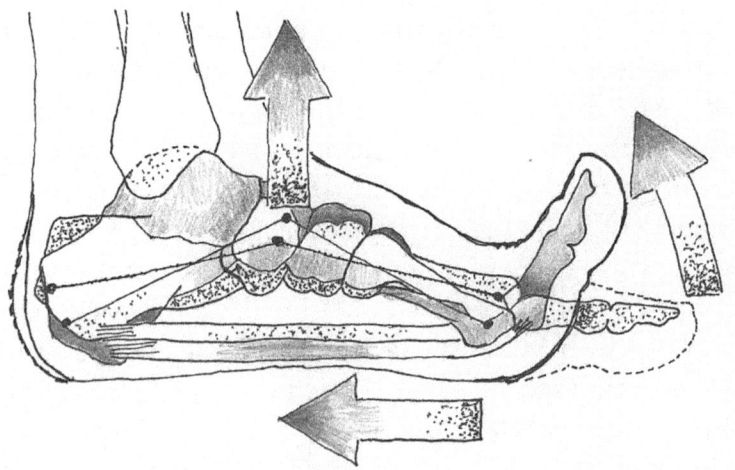

Figure 9. Windlass Effect – with elevation (or dorsiflexion) of the great toe the relatively inflexible plantar fascia causes the longitudinal arch to rise and shorten. This action is repeated with toe-off but also with heel strike. Problems can arise when pronation is "too much, too soon, too fast" and when the talo-navicular-cuneiform joint complex becomes locked.

it a rigid lever. When is the toe dorsiflexed? In the gait cycle this happens twice. With heel strike the toe is up. Most people don't know this because shoes can cover the big toe, but watch someone walk in sandals or bare footed and you'll see the great toe elevate on heel strike.

By "locking" the foot we create a rigid lever. A rigid lever is a poor shock absorber but helps transfer the forces of ground contact (4-7x body weight with running) up the leg to the thigh and rear end muscles, easily the largest muscle groups in the body. Those large muscles help dissipate the force.

The second time the foot supinates in the gait cycle is at toe-off, when we push against the ground and the toe loses contact with the ground. The big toe dorsiflexes, the foot becomes a rigid lever and the forceful contraction of the gastroc soleus complex propels the body forward. You have done this a million times.

The foot pronates (Fig. 10) when one is in mid-stance. Here the foot is the mobile adapter. What does that mean? It acts as a balancer and should help maintain the body's forward momentum, but this is not always the case. I'm sure that is why, at least in part, pronation is frequently seen as a "bad" thing. In truth pronation is normal and necessary. It becomes "bad" when it happens too fast, too early in the gait cycle or lasts too long. Any one of these conditions would more accurately describe pathologic pronation.

It is worth noting how pronation can happen "too fast." As the foot makes ground contact at heel strike (as a rigid lever) and moves towards mid-stance the foot must make a transition from the rigid lever to mobile adapter. The middle portion of the foot unlocks and allows this transition to take place. If the muscles that control the velocity of

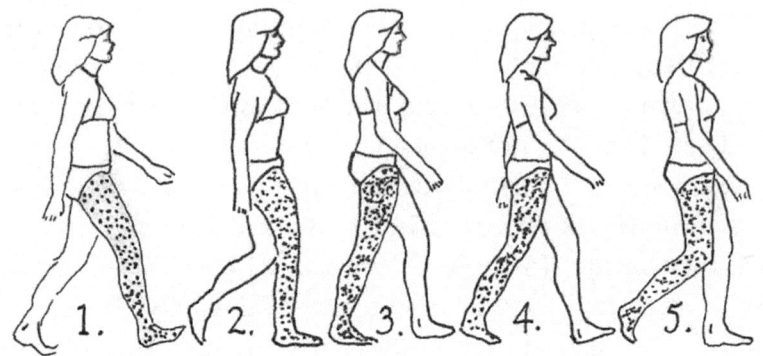

Figure 10. Foot pronation and supination in gait (descriptions are for "black" leg)
1. Heel strike, foot supinated, rigid lever
2. Early mid-stance, foot pronated, mobile adapter
3. Late mid-stance, foot pronated, mobile adapter
4. Early toe-off, foot supinated, rigid lever
5. Toe-off, foot supinated, rigid lever

mid-foot pronation are weak, fatigued or uncoordinated the foot will essentially "flop" into mid-stance.

This flop produces a tremendous stress on the tissues that control this action, notably the posterior tibialis muscle (PT). The PT's tendons stretch out like tentacles and there are between 7-9 insertion sites on the sole of the foot. This flopping action completed in a "too fast," uncoordinated manner can strain the PT leading to posterior tibial tendonitis or what is commonly termed shin splints.

But even with a better understanding of pronation and supination why are these concepts important for a runner? There are actually several reasons, any one of which could have consequences on performance step by step.

In December 2005 and 2006 I was asked to present at the USATF's High Performance Summit on Improving

Distance Running in America. The crux of my two presentations was that if one could decrease one's ground contact time (the time of each foot strike) by 1/100th of a second that would improve a miler's time by 7-8 seconds, a 5k runner by 20-24 seconds and a marathoner by over 3 minutes. All significant improvements simply by getting the foot off the ground more quickly.

How long is 1/100th of a second? To blink your eyes takes 14/100ths of a second and to clap your hands on command takes about 20/100ths so we are talking about an amount of time that is essentially incomparable to any other human action. So how do we improve this?

The answer is to improve one's balance. The subtalar joint in the foot (between the talus and calcaneus) can move in three planes of motion—forward and backward, side to side and at a designated angle. Remember during mid-stance the foot acts as a mobile adapter. As the body passes through this plane the foot attempts to maintain forward momentum. But what if there is a "quiver?" Some unwanted or non-productive side to side motion? What if this "quiver" happens every step? 1/100th, 2/100ths, 3/100ths, etc., all those "quivers" add up. They also mean longer or poorer ground contact times which adds up to slower races and slower racers.

Balance is coordination in its purest sense. If we can better train the balance sense to decrease ground contact times this will also have a direct effect on two other important concepts in running—shock absorption and force generation.

Remember that with heel strike force is transferred to the larger leg muscles. Also recall that pathologic pronation is too much, too soon or too long. If the foot has a poor balance sense (i.e. it is uncoordinated) the shock of ground contact will not be transferred as efficiently to the larger muscles. Why is this a problem? This instability on a microscopic level causes tearing of tissues. Repeated 1000s of times can lead to muscle or tendon injuries. What is the bane of many distance runners? Shin splints, Achilles problems or calf muscle pulls all of which can be directly traced to improper shock absorption due to a poorly coordinated foot.

The second problem is force generation. If the foot moves from mid-stance to toe-off and there is a "quiver" that quiver is dissipation of force. What that translates into is a loss of power or loss of drive. Regardless, the result is the same—there will be slower times and decreased directed force because of the quiver. If you would like to test yourself simply stand on one foot for 30 to 60 seconds. At some point you will begin to fatigue and feel the quiver at your subtalar joint. That is the place to lose force, 1/100th here, 1/100th there, it all adds up.

The final consideration is what is called the closed kinetic chain of the lower extremity.

This helps explain the domino effect pronation has on the knee, hip, sacroiliac joint and lumbar spine. Pathologic pronation (too much, too soon, too fast) or any in-coordination in the action of the leg can cause poor shock absorption, decreased force generation or an increase in ground contact times which may ultimately transfer into injury or slower performance.

Figure 11 neatly illustrates the series of events that happen with foot pronation. Everything begins as the foot moves into mid-stance—the head of the talus drops (A) down, anterior and medially. This inward rotation drags along the shin which in turn drags along the femur (B) (both internally rotate). There is a lengthening stretch to

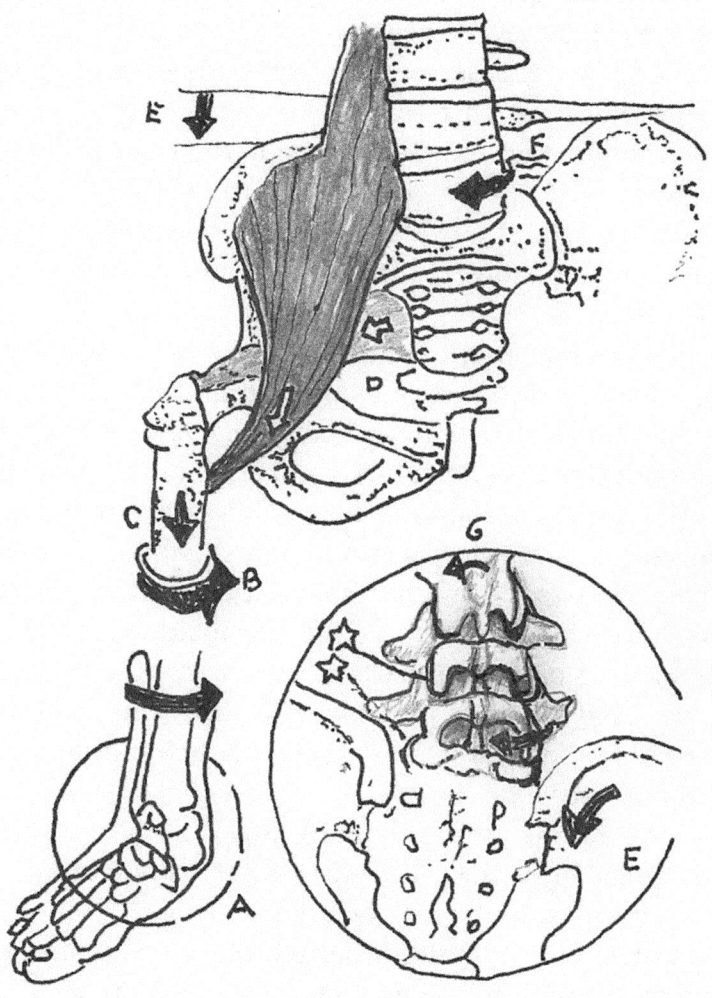

Figure 11. Closed Kinetic Chain of Lower Extremity
A. Longitudinal arch drops "down, anterior and medially"
B. Tibia leads femur in internal rotation
C. Femur drops inferiorly
D. Eccentric stretch to iliopsoas and piriformis
E. Ilia rotates posteriorly
F. L5 lumbar body rotates into right rotation
G. "Reactive" scoliosis into left lateral flexion
   "stars" – facet joints check further lumbar body rotation

both the piriformis and psoas muscles (D). These muscles are critical to pelvic movement and stabilization.

The pelvis tilts backward which causes the sacrum to tilt on one side. This creates an uneven surface for the lowest lumbar vertebrae L5 causing rotation (F) which in turn rotates the vertebrae above creating what is called a reactive scoliosis (G). Finally, the check joints or facet joints block further rotation (stars) but may be jammed together.

Pronation lasting too long, happening too soon or too fast can cause loss of force generation and increased ground contact times. An additional concern could be injuries at the ankle, knee (ligament, IT Band or meniscus problems), the hip (snapping hip syndrome, bursitis, tendonitis), SI joint sprain or the lumbar spine (facet jamming, disc injury or muscle strain). Another one of the my major points in Las Vegas was that balance and coordination are the most important skills of a successful distance runner.

No doubt some are wondering why pathologic supination has not been detailed. Pathologic supination, although possible, is rare. I've seen the number 2% of the population used frequently. So while it can happen, pathologic pronation (60-90% of the population) is a much more common problem.

So what can be done about all this? Actually there are several simple solutions that both address and solve any number of the aforementioned problems. The first solution is to strengthen the foot with foot drills. If you were to Google my name you can find a boot-legged article detailing the foot drills and reasons for doing them *daily*.

Secondly, do some balance work. A balance board is nice but one can significantly improve one's balance sense by simply standing on one foot for 60-90 seconds daily. Try to stand "still" and note how long it takes for the "quiver" to happen. With practice that time should lengthen.

Thirdly consider an orthotic. I will admit an orthotic is a crutch for the foot but the relentless assault of hard level floors, gravity and 1000s of running ground contacts serve to promote pathologic pronation and foot strain. Orthotics are a simple and effective remedy. Any number of healthcare providers can adequately service your needs here—podiatrists, chiropractors or pedorthists—ask around.

Finally, watch your shoes. Modern shoes represent a soft cast for the foot which leads to muscular atrophy. I am not a proponent of barefoot running but I am a proponent of a strong foot. A good shoe should protect the foot from ground surfaces, not restrict the foot from movement, similar to a glove for the hand. Think about it.

So while pronation and supination may still be seen as the foot turning this way or that hopefully you will appreciate that there is more to pronation and supination than simple ankle movements. Foot strike is really central to the activities of a runner and a clear understanding of that import can only serve to make one's training and practice planning more effective and one's competitive performances more rewarding.

Shin Splints

Back in the 90s a study was done in the Seattle area that concluded that high school girls cross country was the most "dangerous" high school sport, ahead of football, wrestling and cheerleading. That conclusion was drawn from the fact that high school girls cross country had the highest injury rate. The combination of five-mile runs, an unconditioned foot and hard pavements are the recipe for foreleg problems. The most common foreleg problem is the shin splint.

If you are new to the sport or even a seasoned veteran, it would be a rare group training run where somebody doesn't start to complain about their "shin splints." The true rookies may wonder where their shin splints came from and if they will ever go away. Shin splints will go away with time, some rest and a sensible resumption plan for training. The best treatment is to prevent shin splints in the first place.

Shin splints are really a "garbage can" term to describe any pain associated with the shin or tibia of the foreleg. More descriptive terms include tendinitis of one of the foreleg muscles, microstress fractures of the tibia or muscular dysfunction in the form of myofascial trigger points. Each diagnosis is the result of the breaking of the "weak link" of the closed kinetic chain of the leg.

Why do shin splints develop in the first place? The umbrella answer is that the body is not prepared for the stresses placed upon it. Running is a ground contact sport. Each foot strike can generate 4-7x the force of body weight (or more) with ground contact. This is repeated a thousand times per mile, mile after mile. The elasticity of our tissues has limits. Weak or poorly conditioned muscles makes the force of ground contact all the more forceful.

Poor running mechanics can also contribute to developing shin splints. Excessive or pathological pronation (where the arch drops excessively in the weight bearing mid-stance) can begin to strain the muscles and tendons that run from the shin to the foot.

Tight, inelastic muscles due to fatigue or muscles that have been poorly warmed up may lead to shin splints. This has to do with the decreased range of motion the muscle has. The daily run and ground reaction forces are the same whether one is "stretched out" or tight. The problem is that ground contact can be more damaging when one is tight.

Exactly what causes the pain with shin splints? The shin splint pain is most often described as "vague." Muscles are attached to roughened areas of bones by tendenous fibers. If these fibers are continually tugged on, they begin to tear. The tearing produces pain. Vague pain is characteristic of generalized tears while sharp pains indicate a larger tear commonly called the muscle pull.

If the shin splints are more common in a poorly conditioned athlete whose newfound enthusiasm for the sport has bested their good sense the solution may seem simple—take it easy. That advice would decrease the pain but do little to solve the problem.

While a more sensible training strategy would be in order the true solution to the problem would be to spend time properly conditioning the foot. Improvement of the strength of the foot will increase the foot's proprioceptive input to the brain and improve balance sense, both combining to make each individual foot strike less stressful.

How does one strengthen the foot? The problem here is that the largest muscle in the foot is not much larger that one's thumb. There is not much muscle to work with. None the less the use of ankle circles and foot drills will help tremendously.

Ankle circles can simply be done in a clockwise and counterclockwise direction. The foot drills should be done in one's bare feet. Walk 25m on the outside of the foot, inside of the foot, toeing in and out and walking backwards on the toes. After putting the shoes back on walk 25m on the heels. These should be done daily.

The use of a balance board will also help strengthen the small intrinsic muscles of the foot and improve the proprioception to the brain. The simplest balance board is to take a 12" by 16" piece of plywood and attach a 2"x 2" wood strip down the center of the board. The use of a balance board for 30 seconds a day will greatly help one's balance on the foot.

A variation is to stand on one leg in single support for 60 seconds. This will challenge the nerve pathways and over the course of 2-3 weeks one can expect to see a significant improvement in one's balance.

Use of a leg extension machine will strengthen the quad and give a better shock absorber, again lessening the stress of ground contact. Therapeutic squats, with the feet shoulder width apart and lowering the butt until the thigh is parallel to the floor will strengthen the gluts which are another important shock absorber. Strong gluts also greatly aid the overall running action.

A final option for treating shin splints is to get an orthotic for the foot. An orthotic will control how much pronation the foot goes through as one moves through the mid-stance of gait. Orthotics support the arch and prevent downward drop of two bones, the head of the talus and the navicular. The dropping of these two bones begins a chain reaction of twisting and pulling all the way to the hip and low back.

Shoes can also contribute to the muscular strain of the foreleg. If the outer sole of the shoe is too stiff the toes and mid-foot cannot move properly as the foot makes ground contact. In truth, the shoe is stronger than the foot. This transfers the shock of ground contact from the foot to the shin helping to create the shin splint.

The solution to the problem is to fold the shoe along the metatarsal crease (where the toes contact the foot) and leave the shoe in that position over night. This will give added forefoot flexibility to the shoe.

Shin splints are one of the nuisance injuries all runners face at sometime in their career. As with most nuisance injuries time spent daily on preventive measures will greatly decrease the incidence of shin splints. Strengthening and improving the balance sense of the foot with the six-foot drills and use of a balance board will help.

Folding the shoe at the toe crease and possibly the use of an orthotic may be indicated.

Ultimately, anything that can improve the shock absorption ability of the leg will help to decrease the shock of ground contact for each step of the 1000s run each training week.

Sports Psychology

A chance encounter at a discount bookstore led to one of the most useful sports psychology books I have ever read. Backed by extensive surveys and loaded with suggestions for practical application the GolfPsyche program easily transfers to track and field.

I have always had a fascination with sports psychology. I can trace it back to my earliest high school days when *Track and Field News* advertised a book called *Problem Athletes and How to Handle Them* by a guy named Tutko. Not that I was a problem athlete, and in truth I never bought the book but what fascinated me was that there was a potential positive solution to dealing with how people act.

As I got into coaching I came to realize that the behaviors of my athletes could either greatly enhance their performance or severely detract from it. The commitment to agreed upon team rules and personal behaviors greatly clarified for all what were the expectations for one to be "on the team." I should add that this included my personal behavior also.

The next great revelation I had in this area was the role that self-esteem played in one's athletic development. By this time sports psychology was becoming a recognized discipline by many. Although I was more interested in things such as visualization and other mental preparation techniques I distinctly remember being disappointed by one clinician with his emphasis on the importance of self-esteem.

But I had the patience to give this concept a chance in terms of observation and application and very quickly I came to see that the "problem athletes" I coached in the past and the ones I was currently struggling to coach all had self-esteem issues. It was a moment of great enlightenment when I realized that the "how to handle them" was to create a coaching environment that in ways great and small conscientiously and consistently fostered individual respect and promoted self-esteem.

And that all worked to an extent, but I was constantly left with the feeling that there was something "more" and that my team's training environment could be made more complete.

Several years ago while shopping in a discount bookstore I happened upon a book called, *The 8 Traits of Championship Golfers* for $2.99. My father was a professional golfer. In truth I am a mediocre golfer at best but I feel because of him that I have a pretty good fundamental understanding of the game. The price was right, I bought the book and it sat on my bookshelf for over a year.

It was a rainy weekend with no big plans when I scanned the shelf, thought I'd give the book 20 pages and then go on to something else. I was sold by page 10.

What the authors, founders of the GolfPsyche sports psychology program had done was a psychological inventory of the top 300 professional golfers of the PGA and LPGA. They even named names—Tiger Woods, Davis Love and many others who are weekly showcased on television. When they tested these golfers they found that eight traits were identified repeatedly as having a critical role in the performance of the golfer. And then they used the rest of the book to test the reader on their strengths and weaknesses with regard to the eight traits, prescribe behaviors or thought patterns to capitalize on one's profile or improve areas of weakness.

It seems like I underlined half the book. Golfers are very much like track and field athletes. They perform individually and rely on themselves for their successes and generally have only themselves to blame for their shortcomings. I wrote down my notes from the book and ended up with 12 handwritten pages.

The eight traits that champions share are: focus, abstract thinking, emotional stability, dominance, tough mindedness, confidence, self-sufficiency and optimal arousal. One of the important concepts put forth is that the traits compliment or synergistically re-enforce each other and that they are part of a formula. The other major concepts were those of content—what to think; and process—how to think. Detailed below is a synopsis of the eight traits, their importance and suggestions for development.

I. Focus

There are three components to successful focus—the fact that it requires a strong mental routine (the how and what you think), the fact that you can only focus on one thing at a time (trying to do more dilutes focus) and the fact that one must learn to "turn on and turn off" focus in that heightened mental focus leads to mental exhaustion. Heightened mental focus is one of the greatest challenges to higher level golf.

All emotional reactions—hope, fear, anticipation, etc. widen one's focus. The challenge comes to stay in the "here and now." Focus is easier for introverts than extroverts. It is easier in reaction sports (basketball, soccer, baseball) than deliberation sports (golf, rifle, billiards) where downtime between "plays" can allow for a widened focus.

Focus can be a challenge if you are too smart (you think too much), too friendly (other directed), too tense (causing your mind to race) or too relaxed (mind wanders). Signs of poor focus include: "choking" when playing well or play has meaning. Mental exhaustion following play (indicating the need to learn how to turn on/off focus) or focus that improves in difficult situations.

Exercises to strengthen one's focus:
1. focus on process, not outcome
2. develop a consistent mental approach or ritual
3. refuse to waiver from mental routine
4. practice staying in the "here and now"

II. Abstract Thinking

Abstract thinking involves the athlete's ability to analyze a situation, creatively problem solve and learn and adapt to different situations. Athletes who excel in this area are seen as fast learners. Basic to successful abstract thinking is thought management—controlling the thoughts of one's mind.

Why do some people have trouble controlling their thoughts? For some there is a lack of personal discipline, they are unorganized. Some lack confidence as evidenced with second-guessing or lack of commitment towards goals. Some react emotionally with a widened focus that allows for irrational reactions. There can also be those that are over coached, not self-sufficient and dependent on others for direction. And other factors such as drugs, illness, injury, fatigue or personal problems can all negatively affect thought management.

One must learn to categorize thoughts into allowed versus non-allowed thoughts. Non-allowed thoughts include: anticipation, negative self-talk, outcome thinking, mind reading (or attempting to mind read) and self-critical thinking. In contrast allowed thoughts include: review of past successes, positive compliments, music—actual or replaying a song in one's head, object meditation (to shift focus during off times) and attention to one's posture.

Exercises to strengthen one's abstract thinking:
1. develop good mental routines or scripts for play
2. learn to regulate allowed thoughts
3. develop a list of allowed thoughts

III. Emotional Stability

Emotional stability affects all eight traits. Emotions give meaning, passion and purpose to events and can drive the desire to improve. But emotional extremes can lead to anger, fear, or insecurity on one hand and over excitement, anticipation and once again fear at the other extreme.

Challenges to emotional stability include: expectations (outcome thinking), perfectionism, mental fatigue, unhealthy body chemistries affected by poor nutrition in combination with negative emotional states such as anger, fear or anxiety.

One of the keys to emotional stability and the whole GolfPsyche program is the differentiation between process and outcome thinking. Before success is an outcome it is a process. The athlete can create the process. Fundamentals should be continually reviewed and applied.

Process goals may include: staying with the game plan, walking with confidence, visualization of actions, looking for the good and defining immediate targets or goals.

Exercises to strengthen one's emotional stability include:
1. practice process thinking
2. work to maintain a healthy lifestyle
3. program adequate daily rest
4. setting aside two hours each week to pursue personal interests

IV. Dominance

Dominance is the balance between assertiveness (making things happen) and patience (letting things happen). Dominance is a combination of calculated risk combined with maximizing one's personal skills and adherence to plans. To a degree dominance includes stubbornness.

Dominance can cause extremes of behaviors (anger, frustration or withdrawal), loss of confidence can lead to passive play and excessive tension can cause one to become too aggressive or too submissive.

To positively manage dominance it is recommended one develop a game plan. The game plan would be part of the previously mentioned process thinking and include a critical assessment of one's strengths and weaknesses, an inventory of one's skills and an avoidance of emotional or ego centered plans.

Exercises to strengthen one's dominance:
1. Pre-set your game plan and stick with it.
2. Create a real or imagined foe to spur one's self on
3. Challenge yourself to perform with excellence in all actions
4. Challenge your competition with your best efforts.

V. Tough Mindedness

Tough mindedness requires one to be emotionally uninvolved with what others are thinking, feeling or doing while one is competing. It is important one emphasize tough mindedness while competing. Tough-minded people keep thoughts simple, emotions even and focus narrow.

The opposite of the tough-minded competitor is the tender minded one. The tough- minded individual can channel their thoughts and efforts in a selfish, indifferent way removed from the needs of others. The tender minded athlete will be emotionally involved, thoughtful and compassionate towards others. While these are certainly admirable traits in a friend or spouse they do not allow for the necessary aggressiveness and dominance required for sport.

Tough minded athletes have the ability to stop non-productive thoughts and maintain or quickly regain focus to the task at hand. A tough-minded athlete would be able to adeptly apply GolfPsyche's eight traits of a champion.

Exercises to develop one dominance:
1. develop cue words or phrases that clearly define one's focus or instantly helps refocus:
    - It's my time!
    - I can do this!
    - Think process

- Now!
- Bring it on!
- I'm strong, I'm fast, I'm confident

VI. Self Sufficiency

Self-sufficiency is one's ability to make difficult decisions. As one's involvement and sophistication in any sport grows the number of potential options or solutions can become overwhelming. This can create an "analysis paralysis" which can be crippling to performance. The champion is one who can quickly make decisions and is committed to them once they are made.

Childhood rearing plays a significant role in self-sufficiency. Highly self-sufficient individuals come from secure environments, were not "over protected," were encouraged with healthy initiative and had opportunities to express their free will. Low self sufficiency athletes have a group orientation, had indulging parents, lack independence and are needy and tend to have trouble with solo sports.

Excessive self-sufficiency can be a double-edged sword. The strong need to resolve one's own problems may lead to burying issues or denial rather than bringing them to resolution. Tense situations coupled with fatigue or heightened emotional states can also decrease one's effective self-reliance.

Exercises to strengthen one's self reliance:
1. learn to trust one's first impressions and don't second guess self
2. be decisive in all actions
3. practice focus, particularly on one's allowed, productive thoughts

VII. Confidence

Confidence is one of the keys to success in everything we do. Confidence is the way we think about ourselves and is broken down into personal confidence and performance confidence.

Personal confidence is a mostly learned behavior. It is a combination of respect for yourself, belief in yourself and belief in one's skills. Champions possess a level of confidence above that of the average person. They dwell on strengths and things they can control. They refuse to allow self doubts and other limiting thoughts dwell in their consciousness. Their focus is on process, the "how to" rather than another athlete's performance.

Low confidence people dwell on personal weaknesses, get involved in things they cannot control, evidence self-doubt and second guessing, worry about poor results, don't learn well from mistakes and think about what they don't want to happen.

Exercises to strengthen one's self-confidence include:
1. affirmations—compliments you bestow on yourself
2. thought checks—maintenance of thoughts that are positive and productive
3. avoidance of mind reading—worry and focus on what others are thinking
4. "all or nothing" thinking—where negatives dominate positives
5. magnification—dramatic, negative deductions
6. defensiveness—taking situations and events personally

Performance confidence is faith in one's mental skills, mechanics of performance, equipment, preparation and coaching. Techniques should be coached in practice, coach confidence on game days.

Exercises to develop performance confidence:
1. use opportunities to compliment oneself and one's performance
2. create challenges or opportunities to develop one's confidence
3. objectively rate one's progress

VIII. Optimal Arousal

Optimal arousal is a state of "good tension" where focus, willfulness, directed energy and process thinking are all actively managed. Under arousal may be the result of a weak commitment, poor mental focus or boredom. Over arousal may result from abandonment of one's game plan, outcome thinking or focus on non-allowed, unproductive thoughts.

Under arousal can be counteracted by exercise, goal setting or raising the stakes (such as self-gambling). Over arousal can be neutralized by slow, deep breathing (four breaths per minute), scanning the body for tension, relaxation techniques and thought checks to focus or refocus mental energy. Time management, scripting competition circumstances and maintenance of personal balance in career, family, diet, etc. all contribute to optimal arousal.

Exercises to develop optimal arousal:
1. identify thoughts and actions that contribute to reaching optimal arousal in a programmed manner
2. learn to identify optimal arousal states
3. focus on process, not outcome.

Stellar athletic performance is the result of many factors, not the least of which is one's mindset. What the GolfPsyche program presents are eight tested traits that individually and in combination create an internal environment that allows one to compete fearlessly and methodically yet not recklessly.

While fundamental concepts such as a positive mental attitude (look for the good, expect the best), personal responsibility (I can do this, self-reliance) and personal discipline (make it happen, be on time) underpin any athlete's success the application of the eight traits detailed above will further develop the athlete's coping and management skills so that competition truly becomes a test of one's potential.

The Athletic Triage Model

The Athletic Triage Model was my solution to David Oja's problem of how to provide healthcare services for the Syracuse Festival of Races. Ultimately this became my thesis topic for my master's in communication at Ithaca College.

Sports participation can be divided into four categories—fundamental development, fitness-based actions, performance-based competitions and pre-hab or rehabilitation work. The first three are pretty straight forward. The first two generate little argument. Pre-hab prevents rehab. But while few get involved in sport simply with the goal of getting hurt and rehabbed, hurt happens.

Rehabilitation is dictionary defined as the process of restoring one who has been ill or injured to a pre-injury state. While the goal of athletic participation is not to pursue rehabilitation any athlete, regardless of the level or training background, faces increasing odds that they will suffer some form of injury due to chronic overuse or direct trauma the longer they participate in a given activity. And rehabilitation is the road back.

Traditionally athletic healthcare or sports medicine has been divided into two portals of entry—care for acute, non-life threatening injuries or treatment for traumatic life threatening injuries. While there are any number of health professionals who could deliver care within this model routinely it is the athletic trainer/orthopedist for the non-life threatening/acute care treatment and the emergency medical technician/medical doctor for the life support care. Together these professionals neatly cover this portion of the injury and illness spectrum.

Whichever practitioner is chosen the care is delivered "after the fact." An injury has happened, and care is sought. Athletic healthcare in this means follows the Reactive Care Model; care is given in reaction to an injury.

Most would agree the Reactive Care Model (Diagram 4) is important and necessary if only from a liability standpoint. And for many high school, college and weekend warriors this is the type of care they are given should they become injured.

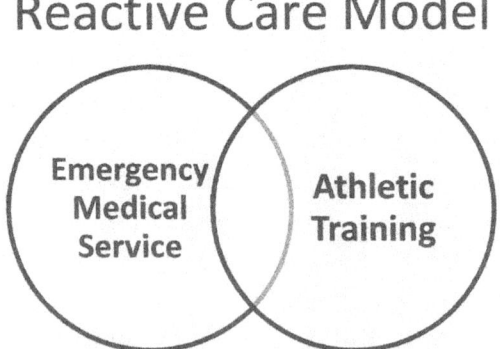

Diagram 4. Traditional Sports Medicine follows the Reactive Care Model. Emergency medical services is for life support. Athletic training is for acute, non-life-threatening care. Overlap represents first aid and CPR.

The problem with the Reactive Care Model is that it only accommodates patients that have an injury or presenting complaint. What about the athlete that gets a massage before a competition? Why are they getting a massage? Most would answer "it feels good" or they "feel better" following the massage. Ask them if they are hurt and the answer is probably, "No." Is this reactive care? No. Is it a form of healthcare? Yes, it promotes health.

The same goes for chiropractic care. Many athletes like to be adjusted prior to a competition. Why? Many feel looser, note an increased range of motion and ease of movement. Are they hurt? Generally, no. Another group prefers to get care following a competition because it helps them recover. Both treatments are not used reactively (after an injury) but proactively—as a means to either compete better or recover faster. The big problem is that within the Reactive Care Model there is no place, no "fit" for either of these proactive therapies (chiropractic or massage).

Since 1999 I have coordinated the Sports Outreach Program at two different chiropractic colleges. At this writing we have provided complimentary chiropractic care at close to 150 events (the number eventually topped 250). These events include many of the marquee track and field meets, road races and triathlon competitions on the East Coast including: Freihofer's *Run For Women*, Utica's *Boilermaker*, the *IC4A Cross Country Championships*, several meets at the Armory including the *National Scholastic Championships*, the *Musselman Triathlon* and we even traveled to Barbados in 2003 for the *Pan Am Junior Track and Field Championships*. While the meet list is impressive our patients have included any number of national champions, Olympic medalists and even world record holders.

We have conducted two patient satisfaction surveys following care at the 2004 Freihofer's *Run For Women* and the 2005 *Head of the Fish Regatta* in Saratoga. Each survey asked 15 questions one of which was, "How did you feel following treatment?" with a list of 18 possible answers, space for write-in answers not listed and the direction to "circle all that apply."

The results were strikingly similar even though the two survey samples were significantly different in age profile and sex. At the Fish 94% of the respondents were aged 29 or less and males outnumbered females 71 to 63. At Freihofer's 63% of the patients were aged 30-59 and females outnumbered males 126 to 14 (there were four 'no answers'). Chart 1 details the frequency of the top eight responses to the survey question, "How did you feel following treatment?"

Chart 1. How did you feel following treatment?

Run For Women (n=144 respondents)			Head of the Fish (n= 135)		
Loose	104	(72.2%)	Loose	96	(71.1%)
Ease of movement	63	(43.8%)	Better	55	(40.7%)
Increased range of motion	52	(36.1%)	Ease of movement	51	(37.7%)
Better	43	(29.9%)	Less pain	51	(37.7%)
Less pain	42	(29.1%)	Increased range of motion	36	(26.6%)
More aware	36	(25%)	Mood improvement	31	(22.9%)
More energy	31	(21.5%)	More energy	30	(22.2%)
Mood improvement	21	(14.5%)	More aware	29	(21.5%)

But in spite of great patient satisfaction there were acceptance problems with the program in the early days. No doubt there was a real fear that our service was going to supercede or replace the established players of the Reactive Care Model. In fact we were never able to "break through" to certain events because this fear persists—the Empire State Games being a notable example even though

Athletic Triage Model

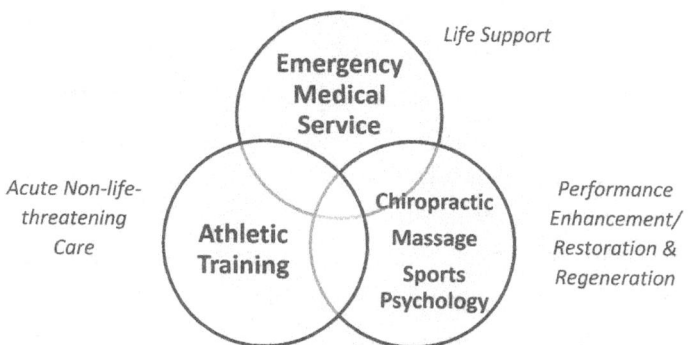

Diagram 5. Athletic Triage Model with the addition of treatments for performance enhancement and restorative or regenerative care to accelerate recovery.

I once served Empire State Games as a coach, competed as an athlete and was a sub-masters gold medalist and record holder. How soon they forget.

For the events currently covered we operate under what I've come to call the Athletic Triage Model (Diagram 5). Within the ATM there is designated space for all the healthcare players to provide care in their area of specialty that compliments, rather than conflicts another healthcare provider's care.

Viewed in this light athletic healthcare takes on a new and distinctly proactive component. In fact, sports training is a proactive activity, an effort to prepare the body for the stresses of athletic competition. Massage therapy and chiropractic care (and sports psychology) compliment the goals of sports training.

This is not lost on America's top track and field programs. Whenever I get introduced to one of these coaches, I hear one of two things—the lament from coaches mired in a Reactive Care Model (Diagram 4) that, "I wish we had access to you guys (chiropractic or massage)." But from the coaches using a proactive care model they ask, "Do you know so and so...?" For the record the teams who are winning have the coaches asking the questions.

Improvement necessitates change. It is truism that works for athletes and society at large. If we keep operating with old models and with blurred focus the dream of success will be achieved by accident rather than by design. On the other hand, the proactive care represented by the Athletic Triage Model (Digram 5) integrated into the larger goals of the general training plan offers increased chances for success due to forward thinking and optimizing utilization of all the healthcare therapies available.

Castor Oil

When I was teaching, I used to assign research topics each semester. Inevitably the lucky student that was assigned castor oil, who had previously never heard of it, would come to my office and ask—"Is this stuff for real? Does this stuff really work? How come I've never heard of it?" At $10 for a 6-month supply versus $10 for a pill, they were starting to see how Big Pharma works.

One of the biggest problems when injured is inflammation at the injured area and what is called the inflammatory response. This is a natural reaction on the part of the body to do a number of things. The swelling of the tissues in and around a joint essentially "splints" the joint restricting movement. Early on this can be important because the decreased movement helps prevent potential further damage to the joint.

But inflammation can also present a problem. Imagine for a second the plumbing has broken in your cellar. Water or sewage leak all over the floor. The to and from flow of the fluids of the house has been disrupted. To remedy the problem the pipe needs to be fixed and the water pumped out, let seep into the ground or possibly left to evaporate.

With most injuries and even stellar performances there is damage to the "plumbing" of the body. Blood vessels, smaller arterioles (from the heart) and veins (to the heart) can sustain damage and spill their contents into the surrounding tissues. The problem is we can't hook-up a sump pump and simply remove the residual swelling.

Anyone who has ever suffered a sprained ankle understands the problem. Early on one of the main goals is to decrease or limit as possible the inflammatory response. The application of the acronym—P-R-I-C-E, pressure, rest, ice, compression and elevation succinctly details the steps one should follow to limit this swelling. The worse the swelling the longer it will take for a full return to activity. Compounding this fact is that the foot is in a dependent position (lower than the heart) and with damaged "plumbing" it is difficult for the body fluids to be removed from the area.

Why is inflammation such a problem? Initially the splinting and limited range of motion may be helpful. It stops you from the offending activity. The problem comes about when a certain type of blood cell called a phagocyte (also known as a macrophage) arrives on the scene. Phagocytes are the tiny garbage men of our body. Their role is to clean up the dead or injured cells. Sometimes they do their job too well and start to damage the cartilage that surrounds the injured joint. If the process is repeated several times over the years it predisposes the joint to an accelerated destruction and the development of degenerative joint disease or osteoarthritis.

As a quick review—inflammation is a natural reaction that initially helps stabilize an injured joint. The problem inflammation causes is when it lasts too long possibly creating long term consequences. A sensible early intervention program begins with the acronym P-R-I-C-E, pressure, rest, ice, compression and elevation.

But not everyone uses the PRICE soon enough or not long enough and then one can develop a chronic low-grade state of inflammation that makes one stiff and reduces the ease of motion. A simple home remedy that will alleviate this swelling is the castor oil pack.

For all the 50 somethings castor oil may have an association with childhood and either constipation or misbehavior. I can only remember getting castor oil once as a child and the histrionics led to alternative treatments in the future. It has been interesting to survey many of my older patients who routinely had castor oil as children and by and large they have lived healthy and carefree lives.

While castor oil is certainly not new its application is simple, and the medicinal effects are profound. Castor oil packs can be made with three simple steps and three readily available ingredients.

Step 1—get some castor oil. Virtually any health food store will have pints for six or seven dollars. (Baar Products if you go on-line)

Step 2—get some white, clean, cotton flannel. Any of the large department or fabric stores will have what you need. You are going to need something you can cut into strips of 3-6" wide and at least two feet long. (an old t-shirt will do)

Step 3—get a box of clingy cellophane wrap (Saran wrap).

Once you have cleaned and dried the flannel you are ready to begin. First saturate the flannel with the castor oil. It should be wet to the touch. Castor oil is greasy and will stain the bed linen so begin the process where a mess can be easily cleaned up.

Secondly, wrap the injured joint or tissue with the castor oil soaked flannel bandage. You don't have to wind the bandage tight, just enough pressure to keep the bandage in place.

The final step is to cover the bandage with a sheet of cellophane wrap. The cellophane wrap will keep the flannel wrap in place and protect the bed linen from stains. Leave the wrap on overnight.

Some people have recommended adding a heating pad, but my personal experience is to leave the heat off.

What can one expect? Results always vary but even patients who don't have profound improvement usually report increased range of motion in the morning. Bruising is often decreased as is the problematic inflammation at the joint.

In truth I have been aware of castor oil for years but never felt the need to give it a try. This past New Year's Eve I was rear ended by a reckless driver and suffered two severely sprained wrists—not a good thing for a chiropractor.

I was desperate for a solution. Coincidentally that December I had read William McGarey's book, *The Oil That Heals* (available from ARE Press), so it was time to put the oil to the test.

For three successive nights I wrapped both wrists in the bandages and left the castor oil packs on overnight. Each morning I felt a little better. That weekend I coordinated the chiropractic services for the Dartmouth Relays and worked three days without problems. I was sold.

How or why does castor oil work? The true mechanism is not fully understood but there are a few things we do know. There is a fatty acid in the castor oil, ricinoleic acid, that is unique. This acid stimulates the lymph flow in the body. The lymph system is a slow-moving sewage canal that transports the dead or diseased cells for excretion.

Facilitation of this transport decreases the inflammation in the area. Decreased inflammation leads to increased ease of movement and a more normal function.

I realize this may all sound too good to be true. I suggest you Google castor oil and research some facts yourself. With 9-10 prescription drugs advertised on the television national news every night it will be a cold day in Iraq before you see either a news story on this treatment or ads touting its efficacy. Nonetheless I am confident that for less than $10. and 10 minutes of your time you will discover a "new" treatment that dates back to the time of Christ.

The Biomotor Skills

*Just exactly what makes an athlete an athlete?
It is the ability to express the five biomotor skills. These five skills are the common denominators of
all athletic activities. The varied contributions
of the individual skills are what makes one sport
differ from another. Now, who is the best
athlete out there? That is another question.*

Gather any mixed group of athletes, add a few beers and it seems inevitable the conversation will soon shift to who is the better athlete. Team sports that require finite skills like basketball have proponents that champion the running, the jumping and the fact that everyone on the floor has to be able to play the game—to a point.

Baseball advocates note that hitting a baseball, especially one traveling 90+ miles per hour is generally considered to be the most difficult feat in sport. Of course, another athlete can counter with the fact that a baseball player's cardiovascular development rivals that of the guy in the press box eating donuts.

And then the runner chimes in to be quickly drowned out with, "Anybody can run!" Which is true, but not everybody can run fast. When I studied in Russia they had a harness set-up that could get anyone to run under 10 seconds for a 100m. While the whole get-up was momentarily exhilarating it also led to some spectacular falls as people's coordination unraveled as they approached the red line. Speed didn't kill that day, but it came pretty close to maiming.

The fact of the matter is that to argue which sport has the greater athletes is akin to arguing which fruit is better. Personal tastes vary, some like apples, some like oranges. It is not really a situation where there is a "right" answer, unless of course you like to argue.

What makes an athlete an athlete is their ability to express what are called the biomotor skills. It is generally accepted there are five biomotor skills that are present to a greater or lesser degree in all sports. It does not matter if we are talking golf or soccer or football or shot putting all the five-biomotor skills are present in each of these disciplines.

With that understanding one can have a more egalitarian appreciation of athletic excellence. Granted some athletes are paid more for what they do than others but when an individual makes it to the top of the rock be it a Super Bowl, World Championship or an Olympics they have distinguished themselves as only a few others ever have.

The five-biomotor skills—speed, strength, endurance, flexibility and the ABC's of agility, balance, coordination and skill are all present to a greater or lesser degree in all sports. You might not think a football lineman or golfer needs endurance but imagine what it must be like having a 20-25 play fourth quarter drive or having to concentrate in 90-degree weather after walking 36 holes and all the marbles depend on your next chip and putt.

The marathon may be all about endurance but come the last 50 yards and it is you and one opponent I'm betting on the one who knows how to sprint.

So you've scanned the list and in check-off fashion you note two things—yes, you can see how the five biomotor skills apply to your sport and secondly, you note that you have stretched or done some speed-type work in the last month. What may come as a surprise is that one should address each of the five-biomotor skills every day.

Wait a minute—speed work every day? How do you combine strength and endurance? At first light that seems like an unrealistic and physically dangerous statement to make.

One of the principles of training and life is that of "use it or lose it." If one does not practice a skill or activity it fades, then vanishes from one's skill inventory. On the other hand if one routinely and consistently practices a skill it becomes more refined, we become better at it. Consider how a musician becomes a musician, a golfer a golfer or a basketball player a basketball player—practice, practice, practice.

For a runner it is equally important to practice the five-biomotor skills on a daily basis. For this to make sense one needs to take a step back and look at the larger training picture. If performance is one's goal (not simply participation) there will be training phases one goes through over the course of a season. The later season training phases usually include a greater emphasis on speed development.

Think back for a second. Traditionally one goes through a protracted period of distance running and the first day of speed work is followed by a day of screaming calves and several down days until the sore legs recover. This is an avoidable problem.

How? By addressing the speed quality every day. I am not recommending repeat 200s or 300s or whatever daily but I am saying to address speed actions daily. How is this done?

Speed actions need to be defined. Sprint biomechanics include a forefoot strike, stepping over the knee with the swing leg and the thigh being parallel to the ground. Arm actions include swinging the hand to the mouth and on the back swing the hand going to the hip or side pocket.

A daily review of "speed actions" may incur 3x25m of skipping with emphasis on a forefoot strike and bringing the thigh parallel to the ground. By reviewing the parts of speed actions or sprinting and challenging the body on a daily basis, "using it" firmly establishes the neurological patterns necessary to sprint and maintains the muscular strength and flexibility necessary to avoid the usual morning after soreness.

Each day's workout should ideally consist of three components—a warm-up, the main focus of the workout and the warm down/conditioning phase. At some point during the course of each day's work the five-biomotor skills should be addressed.

It really does not matter which sport you choose; you still need to drill the five skills. What one needs to determine is which drills are most appropriate for the given sport. Other examples of speed action drills include: fast foot machine gun steps for six to seven seconds, an ankle flick that mimics the plantar flexion of the foot when sprinting or 4-5x 40m stride outs at the end of a practice. Each of these drills addresses a speed quality.

Strength could be practiced by lifting weights, doing push-ups, or sport specific for a runner might be going on a 90 minute to two-hour run. Flexibility would be the traditional stretching, a yoga routine or inclusion of a dynamic movement warm-up with skips and hops or lunge steps.

There are various ways to develop endurance that could include interval, repetition or continuous runs but I also developed secondary endurance by enforcing a "no sit down" rule for practice. Standing is a great endurance quality.

The ABC's could be addressed with a serpentine "snake run" warm-up jog, daily use of a balance board or coordination of arm-leg action in running or skill work with a medicine ball. Understand these are but a few examples and there are countless others. Also each quality is addressed, not belabored. Remember, the use it or lose it maxim, while speed or endurance or strength might not be the focus of a daily workout it is nonetheless a very important component.

Honestly the whole subject gets more complicated when you consider that there can be combinations of skills that need be addressed for one's competitive abilities to become more refined. Speed-strength, speed-endurance or strength-endurance all may have their application but probably are qualities that are better addressed as the main theme of a workout.

So the next time the discussion of Brett Farve, Kobe Bryant or Usain Bolt comes up you'll be better prepared to serve as the voice of reason, not that it will make any difference but at least you'll know, that you know, what you are talking about.

The Hamstrings

Hamstring health is a combination of coordination, balance and strength that combine to create and allow for dynamic stability of the hip. The adductor magnus has a secondary function of hip extension that is commonly ignored by competitive athletes all the way up to the professional ranks. Pre-hab type conditioning can go a long way towards insuring this critical driver in speed and power events.

Most runners or performance-based athletes could identify the hamstring muscles and accurately tell you the function of the muscles that make up the posterior thigh. But in spite of some pedestrian knowledge about these muscles there is a disconnect when it comes to developing strength to the hamstrings or maintaining the health of this muscle group critical for forward movement.

The hamstrings are actually a group of three muscles whose primary role is to extend the hip and secondarily flex the knee. Moving from the inside out are the semimembranosus, semitendonsus and the biceps femoris (Fig. 12). Unbeknownst to most people is that the largest adductor muscle, adductor magnus found on the medial thigh also functions secondarily as a powerful hip extensor. This fact has major implications for strength,

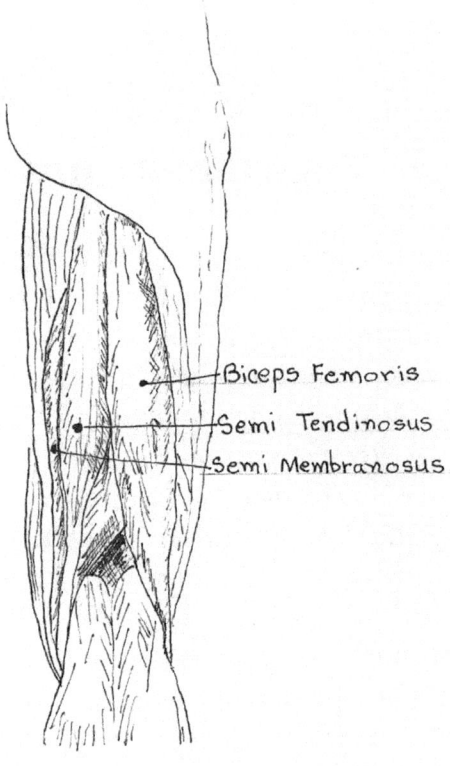

Figure 12. Hamstrings from posterior for right leg

force application and injury occurrence as often times the "groin pull" suffered by many football players is a strain of the undertrained adductor magnus.

The hamstrings are considered to be the fastest muscles in the body. Consider this, a top end sprinter takes about 4.5 strides per second. That means each leg must travel from the thigh being parallel to the ground (Fig. 13) to an extended hip (Fig. 13) 2.25 times per second. By itself that fact might not raise any eyebrows.

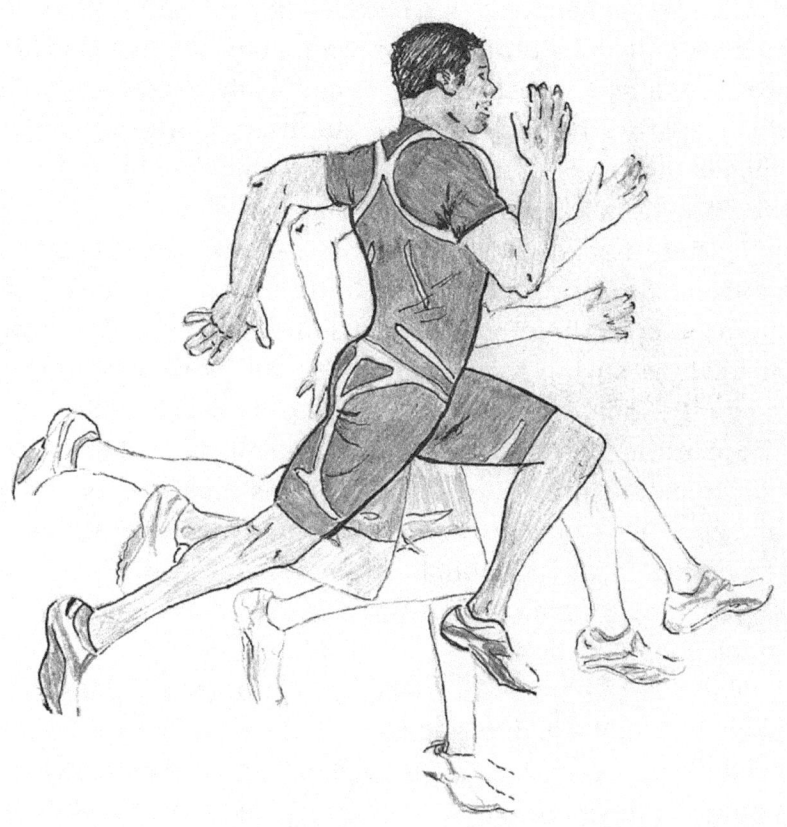

Figure 13. With a red-line efforts the sprinter's hips must cycle through full extension and flexion 4-5x per second while maintaining balance, forward drive, an acceleration pattern, proper technique and force application.

What one must remember is that the moment the thigh is parallel to the ground it is motionless for a fraction of a second. The same is true when the hip is in the extended position. What makes this point amazing is that during this cycle of knee-up to thigh back the leg has reached a velocity of 55 miles per hour. The leg has been sped up to 55mph and slowed down from 55mph. Our muscles and nervous system control both these actions.

Remember that each leg is moving zero mph to 55mph to zero mph 2.25 times per second. Complicating this act is that the body must remain dynamically balanced while the legs drive the body forward. Additionally, the legs must absorb the shock of each step that can be 7-10 times body weight with maximal sprint efforts.

If there is a slight muscular imbalance, asymmetrical motion or incoordination within the system there can be big problems. Understanding this one can appreciate how and why a sprinter can be running full bore and almost instantly, sometimes within one-step crash and burn.

Sprinting and fast running are actions that call for "triple extension" of the leg. What this means is that the hip, knee and ankle push to an extended position to propel the body forward. It could be argued that the great toe also extends (or plantar flexes) but that is generally not given much consideration.

This triple extension is an important point to understand. Were one to poll a random group of runners on how to strengthen the hamstring most would say by doing a hamstring curl on the machine at the local gym. The problem with using a hamstring curl machine is that it makes the muscle strong as a knee flexor, particularly the lower 1/3 of the muscle and the short head of the biceps femoris. Remember sprinting is triple extension, hip extension using the upper 1/3 of the muscle. There is a foundational concept in coaching called specificity of training—you train muscles as you'll use them. Training the hamstring as a knee flexor is a flagrant violation of this principle.

A related controversy is the quad to hamstring strength ratio. Most any physical education student will tell you the correct ratio between the quad and the hamstring should be 3:2. If one can lift 60 pounds with a leg extension (quad muscles) one should train with 40 pounds for the hamstring curl. While this is technically correct it ignores the context in which the hamstring is used in running.

The 3:2 ratio is correct if one is talking about knee rehabilitation, after meniscus or ACL surgery. If we are talking about triple extension the correct ratio becomes 1:1 for knee extension to hip extension.

The adductors also play a critical role in hamstring functionality. Try this simple experiment. From a stand try to touch your toes. Make a mental note of how close you come. Now do a "groin stretch," side to side to stretch out the adductors. Gently go 3-4 times each side. Now try to touch your toes again. No doubt you'll have a 3-4 inch increase in the range of motion of the hip and the hamstrings were not even addressed. One should always do a groin stretch before stretching the hamstrings.

A second experiment illustrates the lack of coordination most runners have between the hamstring and adductors. Lie on your back. Spread your knees apart and for 10-15 seconds bring the knees in and out. Note how jerky and uncoordinated this action is. It begs the question if this action cannot be performed smoothly in an essentially non-weight-bearing situation how will the muscle function in a top end sprint effort?

Strengthening the hamstrings for the demands of fast running can be done several ways. The traditional squat exercise is an excellent start (Fig. 14). Place the feet slightly wider than the shoulders and drop down until the thigh is parallel with the ground. Take care not to lean forward. The kneecap should not move ahead of the toes. This can be done with or without weights and will tone not only the hamstrings but the gluts as well.

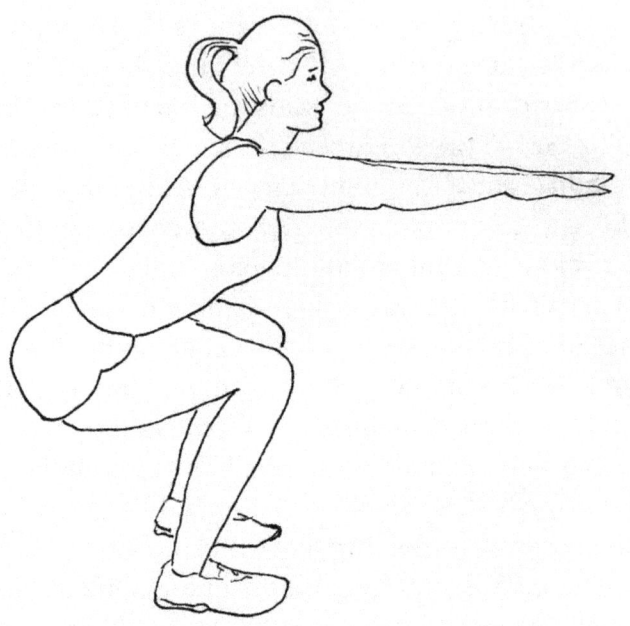

Figure 14. Traditional squat - thigh is parallel to the ground. Note that the kneecap or patella does not move ahead of the great toe.

A second exercise is the lunge step. With the hands on the hips step forward and drop the back knee down to the ground. You can rise up and repeat on the same leg or alternate legs moving down the track or field. It is easy to overdue this exercise so start conservatively with 10 steps and build from there. As fitness improves weights can be added.

A third exercise is a standing hip extension. One needs a "hip extension" machine for this. Keeping the knee straight with the resistance against the posterior thigh sweep the leg backward, extending the hip. This isolates the upper 1/3 of the hamstring and also tones the gluts.

A hip extension machine also allows one to tone the

adductors. By changing body position with the resistance against the inner thigh one can isolate the adductors. Again the goal here is tone as opposed to development. Start conservatively with a light weight and higher rep count.

Hamstring injuries are a common problem for performance sport athletes. Oftentimes they are the result of a faulty training plan. Attention must be given to training the muscle for the exceptional demands it will meet from both a speed and strength perspective. Attention should also be given to the adductor group that works synergistically with the hamstrings. To ignore this reality invites injury as any subtle incoordination can become readily apparent with redline efforts. A deeper understanding of the hamstring is a key to justifying greater preparatory work which will hopefully lead to safer superlative efforts.

The Neti Pot

A stuffy nose, chronic sinus problems or sore throats can all be helped with periodic use of a Neti Pot. It is safe and effective and start to finish takes less than two minutes to do the procedure.

If you take a moment and breathe in through your nose more than likely you'll notice that more air comes in one nostril than the other. If you do this self-check throughout the day you'll note that the nostril that "breathes better" will shift from side to side.

So what is the significance of this? For a runner or really any athlete one of the limiting factors in athletic performance is how much oxygen can be absorbed by the lungs. This is what endurance training is all about, to increase this capacity. Anything that decreases this capacity, like a blocked nasal passage, will subsequently decrease performance.

The nostrils are passages that lead to the sinus cavities. These are hollow areas in the head that are lined with what are called mucous membranes. When one inhales the air passes over the mucous membranes and any impurities in the inhaled air—dust, pollen, mold spores, dandruff, smoke particles cling to the mucous membranes. This is a protective device on the part of the body so that the impurities don't make it to the lungs. In truth this is not a failsafe set-up. Diseases such as coal miners' Black Lung or mesothelioma which asbestos workers suffer from are examples of conditions that develop over a period of years where the concentration of inhalants is greater than the nasal passages' capacity to clean the air.

Masks of all kinds are available from the over the head gas mask for WMD's to the simple cloth dust mask. While neither is perfect they both have their uses, but for an athlete any type of mask becomes impractical.

Athletes, with daily athletic training subject their lungs to increased exposure to foreign particles in that the athlete would take so many more breathes due to their increased work capacity over sedentary individuals.

Problems begin to surface when the sinuses become clogged due to their inability to clean themselves of the foreign substances. Many readers will have experienced seasonal sinus problems during flower pollination periods or in the fall with the molds of decaying leaves. The sinuses swell and occlude the nasal passages leading to a variety of ills ranging from difficulty breathing to headaches.

The simple solution is to head for a pharmacy and purchase some over-the-counter (OTC) nasal spray or nose drops. Generally, if the problem is not terribly serious, these products work well. But what if you are in training for the Olympics or some other high level competition?

Why would the choice of a nasal spray be a consideration? It would matter because many of the OTC products sold to treat simple maladies like clogged sinuses or sore throats would cause one to test positive on a drug test, usually for amphetamines. Goodbye gold.

Regardless of one's intent a positive is a positive and along with it comes public humiliation, loss of status and a stain to one's reputation that will last longer than a bad tattoo. Mistakes are costly and sins of omission are adjudicated just as strictly as sins of commission.

The Neti (sometimes Netti) Pot is a simple non-drug solution for cleaning the sinus cavities. There is probably not a reader who at one time or another has not washed out their mouth with mouthwash or saltwater solution. Millions of dollars are spent annually promoting the perils of bad breath.

What the Neti Pot does is allow one to "wash out" the sinus cavities. I am not sure of the exact origins of this procedure but I'm confident it can be traced to Yogic traditions. When one stops to think for a moment it only makes sense. Men and women routinely clean numerous body cavities, why not the nasal cavities as well?

The Neti Pot is simple to use. The Neti Pot itself is like a small tea pot. They sell ceramic and plastic models. The pot is filled with warm to the touch tap water and between a teaspoon and tablespoon of sea salt dissolved in the warm water.

Step two is to gently insert the spout of the Neti Pot into one nostril, tip the head away and pour the saltwater into the nostril. In truth one's initial attempt may prove a bit gagging as some saltwater drips down the throat. Subsequent uses decrease that feeling. The procedure is repeated in the other nostril and then the nose is blown to clear the passageways.

This simple procedure will open the sinus passages and clean them out of any foreign particles adhering to the serous membranes. A second benefit of the periodic use of the Neti Pot is that this procedure will also help prevent or clear up "sore throats." As most know the sinus passages drain into the throat (postnasal drip) and clearing these passages will remove much of the offensive foreign particles along with creating a postnasal drip of saltwater that serves as a mini-gargle for the throat.

I have used the Neti Pot for years and recommended it to countless patients, usually with very positive results. In 2005 at the World Championships in Helsinki the Neti Pot was all the rage among the American distance runners who suffered head colds. Its use made an immediate and significant difference.

Most health food stores would carry the Neti Pot and the sea salt. As with any healthcare advice self diagnosis and self treatment are not without risk. If symptoms persist past three days seeking professional advice would be a wise decision.

The Stretching Controversy

One would think stretching has been figured out by now...even though this article was written back in 2011 you still will get varying opinions on when to stretch and what to stretch. Discussed are some simple strategies and some resources for those so inclined.

One would think with all the research and scientific advancements that are part and parcel of our daily lives the practice of stretching would not, could not generate any controversy. The fact is, one would be wrong.

It is not that the experts disagree on whether or not one should stretch (most agree) but the controversy is all about when one should stretch and how.

If you watch a dog or cat upon waking they stretch. They appear to have the how and when pattern down. Their routine is to stretch the back and usually the shoulder and hip joints. And then it is on with life.

The problem with humans is we like to complicate things, particularly if one is involved in sport. Surely most would note the increased joint range of motion from something as simple as toe touching. And I am also sure most would question why this is bad.

In truth it is more important to understand why we need to stretch in the first place. Flexibility is one of the five biomotor skills that along with strength, speed, endurance and skill make an athlete an athlete. One of the unique qualities of flexibility is that it is the only non-competitive biomotor skill. One cannot enter a competition for flexibility. Although I have heard that there is lobbying to get competitive yoga in the Olympics.

Nonetheless flexibility serves several critical functions for an athlete. An elastic joint allows for a fuller range of motion which in turn can produce more powerful force application. One can also potentially activate a more forceful stretch reflex (assuming correct technique) which can also aid performance.

Flexibility also pays a critical role in injury prevention. Remember—maximal use is always abuse. The constant starting and stopping of repetitive efforts can lead to the accumulation of microtears to the soft tissues that accumulate over time. What some would dismiss as "age" can be also described as the consequences of this repetitive microtrauma endlessly repeated to an ill prepared joint complex. One's athletic life longevity directly hinges on one's ancillary recovery methods and personal lifestyle, that includes flexibility.

Much of the controversy regarding flexibility revolves around intent. In yoga, for example, the intent is usually relaxation and creation of a meditative state. This can be therapeutic for a number of reasons but if one is involved in an explosive power event such as the 100 meters this type of flexibility would be counter productive. Meditative yoga would have a calming effect on the nervous system, whereas the demands of sprinting call for a heightened state of awareness and an alert nervous system.

This leads to one of the other controversies regarding stretching—how should one stretch before or after a competition? For most stretching is stretching. You assume a position and hold it for a period of time. Some warn about stretching before competition. Most like to feel "loose" before they compete, and they achieve this through stretching. While "looseness" may be dismissed as a psychological quality (it cannot be objectively measured with a meter or machine) most would agree that it is important for an athlete to approach a competition feeling ready, with a heightened state of awareness, however this readiness is achieved.

Use of long, relaxing stretching prior to a competition not only calms the mind but also decreases the responsiveness of the neuro-muscular system. The solution? Short stretches to an end point and back off. This can be repeated 5-7 times. The point here is to improve one's range of motion, ease of movement while not necessarily maximizing one's flexibility. Use of dynamic movements to end range, holding one to two seconds and then backing off—almost that quick.

Post competition stretching is a different story. Most athletes who have made a competitive effort may experience muscle soreness in the coming days. One way to decrease this muscle soreness is to stretch after a competition. After one has done a cool down and the heart rate has approached normal 10-15 minutes of easy stretching can go a long way towards normalizing body functions and decreasing any soreness in the coming days. In this case holding a position 7-10-15 seconds would be recommended with the position repeated several times. An added action that has proven particularly effective is to follow the stretching with 5-10 minutes of cold immersion.

Cold immersion is where one plunges into a tank or pool with water that is usually below 65 degrees Fahrenheit. Although not for the faint of heart this has several therapeutic effects on the body. It temporarily "freezes" the tissues in an elongated position. This allows for greater ease of movement especially combined with the fact that the colder water has an analgesic effect numbing the pain of a superlative effort. The pressure of the water (called hydrostatic pressure) also has the effect of squeezing inflammation out of the traumatized joints which facilitates healing and also aids ease of movement.

But when is enough flexibility enough? You have no doubt made the comparison of yourself and a friend and concluded that he or she is either more or less flexible than you. Are there standards?

In fact a therapist named Gray Cook (*Movement: Functional Movement Systems*, On Target Publishing) has come out with a short list of seven movement postures one should be able to execute that indicate a critical and healthy range of motion for a joint complex. Cook has correlated these movements with balance and symmetric movements of other body parts.

Competitive sport is a series of coordinated movements, not static postures. Due to the repetitive nature of practice and competitions there is a tendency to overdevelop an area of the body due to the demands of the sport. Distance running is essentially a linear activity which erodes one's ability to move laterally. This over development predisposes one to injuries that are characteristic for one's activity.

What Cook has postulated is that the inability to perform his dynamic movements for certain joint complexes provides a strong correlation with the potential for injury to that area of the body. It is a simple analysis but a brilliant observation. What makes this line of thought all the more intriguing is that even the most highly accomplished athletes evidence some, if not many glaring deficiencies. They excel in spite of themselves. Imagine how good (or how long) athletic careers could be if athletes could compete with optimal body symmetry?

One exam that provides a very telling example for most runners is the simple squat. The ability (or inability) to squat down, getting the hips below the knees while keeping the heels flat on the ground tells volumes about one's low back, hip, knee, ankle and foot flexibility. The inability to "sit on the heels" from a stand may indicate either an impending or chronic injury to the plantar fascia, Achilles, gastroc, knee or low back. The quick exam would highlight areas to work on, over a period of weeks, in a post workout flexibility session.

As mentioned in an earlier column Hittleman's *28-Day Guide to Yoga* would be an excellent post-competition habit to acquire. Stretching before? Keep it short and movement oriented. That will allow one to optimize one's range of motion while not unnecessarily maximizing it.

The stretching controversy will not resolve anytime soon due to people's understanding and misunderstandings of anatomy and physiology. But what I have long taught and practiced is to clearly differentiate the stretching that is done before and after an activity. Just as one should train with intention, one should stretch with a specific intention in mind.

Think 145

We have all coached athletes that compete with a degree of mindlessness. This can make for some funny stories as well as some disappointing results. It is the practiced automation of behavior that can provide a pathway or modicum of behavior that can ensure a coach's sanity and allow the athlete to more closely approximate their potential.

It seems to happen with the regularity of a full moon. You flick on the TV and there is a car chase leading the nightly news. The driver seems to break every rule they taught you in driver's ed—high speeds, red lights run, wrong way travel and almost predictably a car crash to end it all. If time allows you get the slo-motion replay that makes one's head shake and spurs a universal thought—what were they thinking?

As it turns out—not much. Scientists have studied this bizarre behavior and found that the adrenalin rush of the chase raises the heart rate to astronomical levels, well above 145 beats per minute. This causes a physiologic reaction in the body where the blood is shunted (redirected) from the cerebral cortex portion of the brain.

The problem is that shunting the blood from the cortex effectively shuts down that area of the brain that includes logical thought, reason and judgment. The shunting of the blood and the loss of these functions fosters a more primitive, simplistic and instinctual "fight or flight" response.

Interestingly the shunting of the blood can affect the chaser as well as the chasee. The surge of adrenalin in the police officer, with a subsequent loss of reason and judgement has been seen as one of the reasons police officers revert to excessive force that has been recorded on dashcams or gone viral on YouTube. Once the heartrate zooms humans begin to exhibit behaviors that are embarrassingly not-so-human.

So what does this have to do with competitive athletics in general or running in particular? Depending on your training philosophy, be it tempo runs, zonal training, intervals or H.I.I.T. one of the goals of each of these methods is to crank the heartrate above 145 beats per minute to get a desired training effect.

Fortunately, in a controlled training environment we don't see people going wild during or after an interval workout but what you might notice is a subtle lack of inhibition that does follow a hard workout or race.

From a spectator's viewpoint one can observe the effects of crossing this 145 heartrate barrier in the later stages of a track race, particularly (but not exclusively) with novices. The runner enters the last lap of a mile and suddenly they take off. He or she has started their kick 60-70 seconds out which proves to be both a distance and pace they cannot maintain leading to stretch drives that are painful to watch.

One would think these runners would "learn from their mistake" but the opposite is often the case. They have developed a pattern (an unthinking one) that although untenable becomes their default pattern which can be difficult, if not an impossible habit to break for both the athlete or coach.

If one truly understands the shunting business and the loss of the higher cognitive functions it no doubt dawns on you that we all become a slave to our lower, instinctual behaviors. While this statement may be generally true it is not necessarily a point of despair.

One of the goals of training is to automate behavior. This means to make certain actions and movements automatic, make them our default mode of movement. This type of action has several advantages. First and foremost, this instinctual movement pattern does not require thinking nor does it require the involvement of the higher processing functions of the cortex.

The advantages of this should be obvious. You get into the later stages of a race, your heart rate begins to skyrocket but tactically you still do the right thing, you compete as opposed to blindly charging ahead at an inopportune time and die in the stretch.

The goal then becomes to develop automatic behaviors. This part is not so simple. It takes forethought, planning and a diligent attention to detail. Fundamental movement patterns such as arm actions, knee lift, foot placement combined with using visual cues (a marking on a track, a tree or rock in cross country) can be used to cue subsequent actions. These actions need to be practiced again and again, day-in and day-out until the desired actions become unconscious. They become the way you move. Think of how Bruce Lee could defend himself with his martial arts discipline.

Concurrent with these deeply engrained movement patterns is the adoption of a training philosophy regarding "training to failure." There is a recurrent, generational thought within the coaching profession that is supported with pithy maxims such as "no-pain, no-gain" and the necessity of giving 110% effort. Unfortunately, these sentiments are often a cover for coaching insecurity or over preparation, ultimately resulting in over-training.

Training to failure is training to fail. When running form, a desired, coordinated movement pattern begins to breakdown one is no longer practicing productive movement skills. One is practicing "bad habits" which in "the heat of the moment" (read this as heart rates above 145 beats per minute) become the patterns that are practiced, learned and used. Therefore, it becomes incumbent that one "practice what you can do, not what you can't," i.e. don't train to failure.

Automatic actions can be learned with forethought, time and practice, practice, practice. Training to failure subverts the process. For the recreational runner this is not much of a concern, but if competitive performance is one's goal attention to this training goal will pay dividends come race day. And if by chance on the day of the meet you see flashing lights in your rearview mirror—pull-over.

Training Theory

Training theory is really about planning your work and working your plan. The ability of a coach or athlete to master this planning ultimately proves to be a tremendous competitive advantage in the short term and will contribute to career longevity in the long term.

In sport, as in life, there is rarely success by accident. Of course there is the lottery but for the vast majority who have achieved any level of accomplishment this has come as the result of energy, effort, and some method or design rather than pure luck.

Training theory as applied to sport is really a complex mix of time management, physiology, rest and recovery, diet and nutrition and a realistic assessment abilities and the setting of goals. This mix needs to be strategically and tactically combined to produce a desired result.

In performance based sport the ability to seamlessly combine these varied skills cannot be emphasized enough. All of this takes time and time is of the essence in sport. In fact the limiting factor in athletic development is not enough time. While that statement may be dismissed as a simple aphorism to the knowing it is a profound truth.

Just as the days of our lives are numbered so are the days of one's athletic career. For the high level athlete the generally accepted time period for competition is 10-12 years. This number can vary depending on multiple factors not the least of which is the nature of the sport.

While it is possible to extend one's career in a team sport by assuming a secondary role individual sport athletes do not have that luxury. In track and field or distance running the athlete is the "team." Their effort is their performance—there is no place to hide.

Modern training theory is based on the work of Hans Selye. Selye was a Canadian endocrinologist who chronicled and popularized the role stress plays in one's daily life. His landmark work, *The Stress of Life* details both the positive and negative affects stress has on humans.

Selye's General Adaptation Syndrome (GAS) curve (Diagram 6) is essentially a pattern of life. At birth we enter the world unable to care for oneself. At the age of reason (about 5 years old) we begin to be able to fend for ourselves. This leads to a period where we thrive through

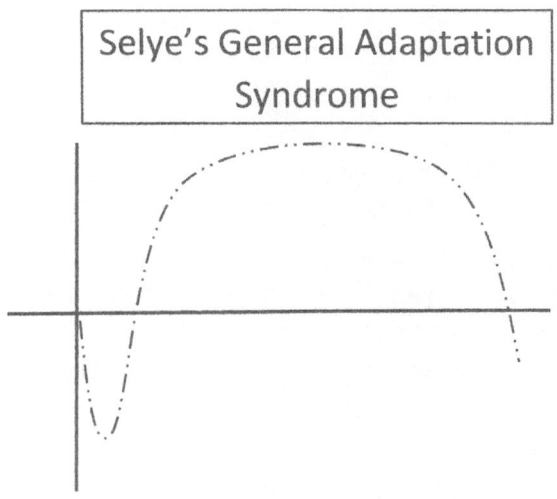

Diagram 6. Selye's classic model of the General Adaption Syndrome cycle

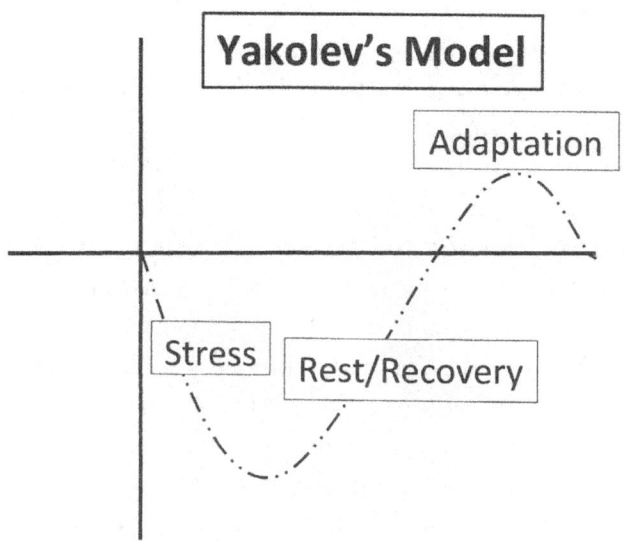

Diagram 7. Yakolev's Model is the adaption of Selye's G.A.S. model to sport. Training is a series of repeated cycles of stress-rest/recovery-adaptation.

adolescence and adulthood. Old age begins a gradual decline that ends in death.

In 1955 Russian physiologists modified Selye's curve to follow the mathematical sine-wave. This has come to be known as Yakolev's Model. (Diagram 7) This stress pattern was modified so that one cycle of the sine wave came to represent a period of time that could in turn represent a workout, weekly pattern, a series of weeks, a season or even a career.

The pattern of the curve can be broken down into three component parts—stress, rest and adaptation. When viewed in this manner the coach or self-coached athlete now has a model from which decisions can be made as to what is the appropriate training plan or means to accomplish long-term future goals.

Although Yakolev's model is simple by design the actual application of the design can become quite complex. Such questions as what gets trained? What gets trained first? How much is enough? How are things sequenced? What does a warm-up count for? While these questions may be beyond the concern or comprehension of the Junior Olympian or outside the scope of concern for the fitness enthusiast they remain central to the performance based athlete.

One must remember that what gets trained are the five biomotor skills—speed, strength, endurance, flexibility and the ABC's of agility, balance, coordination and skill. But simply knowing the ingredients needed to make bread doesn't make one a baker. In training the biomotor skills there is a proper sequencing, combination and benchmarking that are necessary to insure their thorough and complimentary development.

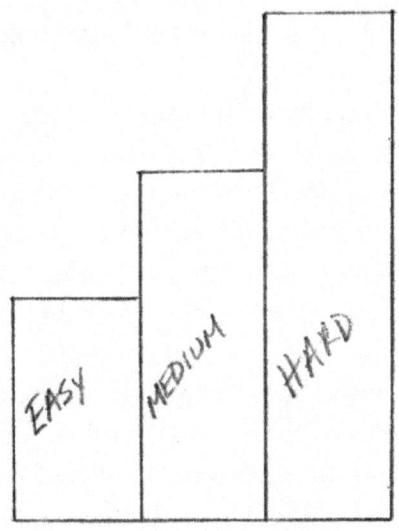

Diagram 8. Suggested cycle of hard-medium and easy days or weeks that represent a fundamental pattern of programmed development.

One of the other critical components of training theory is the cycling of effort with a series of repeated hard, medium and easy days (Diagram 8). This is consistent with Yakolev's model in that the easy days allow one to recover. One needs to remember that all improvement comes while resting and adequate time must be set aside for this. While this truth may seem paradoxical to the novice or obsessive trainer it is either self-evident or something that cannot be ignored by the elite athlete.

Cycling though hard, medium and easy days and weeks of training over a season or career allows the coach to plan, develop and significantly improve the willing athlete. As I better understood, accepted and fully integrated these concepts into my coaching it produced such a coaching advantage, especially at the end of a season, that at times I felt like I had cheated.

The problem many coaches and athletes face is trying to define what constitutes a hard workout, medium workout or easy workout. As a rule of thumb an easy day has been categorized as a day with a 65% effort or less. But 65% of what? A simple answer is the amount of effort it takes to break a sweat, what a good warm-up should do. Then the day is done. For the compulsive individual or chronic over trainer these words are sacrilege.

A medium day is one from which the next day's recovery is not a problem. Hard efforts may be a competition day, a longer distance run, interval workout or any workout that raises the intensity of the heart rate over 160 beats per minute for a sustained period of time. In sum, anything that makes you sore the next day was probably a hard workout.

Other factors that might make a medium workout "hard" could be excessive travel, missing sleep or time zone changes. Emotional upsets can produce extra stress and be seen as stressors that might make a routine workout that much more difficult.

Tactful cycling through hard, medium and easy workouts or weeks of training will help prevent overtraining (OT). OT can be defined as doing too much work and not allowing the body enough time to recover. (Diagram 9) OT eventually results in illness (physiological injury) or physical breakdown (physical injury) to the body. Obviously both are unhealthy stresses but when viewed in the larger context they are problematic because the time spent in illness or injury is time away from growth and development. And remember the limiting factor in athletic development is not enough time.

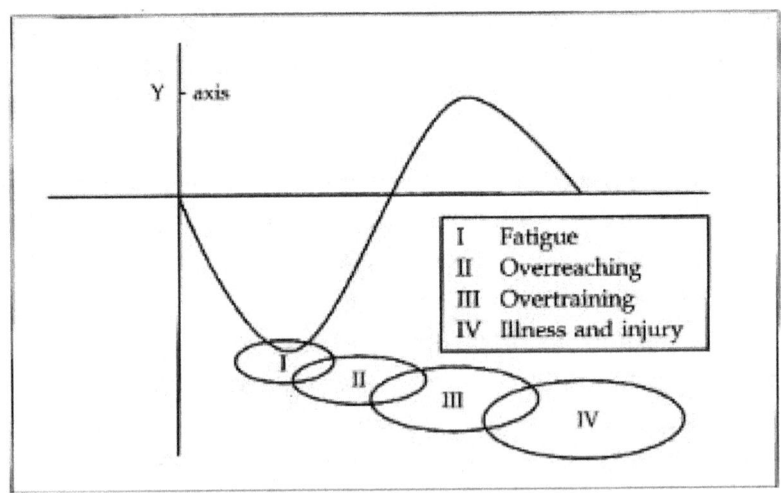

Diagram 9. Yakolev's Model with the progressive nature of I. Fatigue, II. Overreaching, III. Overtraining and IV. Illness/injury. Note the possibility of increased lost training time as the severity of overtraining progresses.

These few paragraphs have only scratched the surface of training theory. Hopefully one can see that all training temporarily compromises the health of an athlete when workout effort and subsequent fatigue drives the athlete to the bottom of the sine wave. If one is allowed proper recovery time there is a rebound effect and the athlete will adapt to the stress of training at a higher level of fitness.

F. Scott Fitzgerald wrote that "brave (wo)men play close to the line." One can see that the continual, self-induced fatigue state of Yakolev's model constantly puts the athlete's health at risk on a daily, weekly and seasonal basis. One's ability to feel the heat of the candle's flame and not get burned is akin to the art of coaching.

The application of training theory is not to predict the future but rather create it. It becomes incumbent that the coach or self-coached athlete train with intention. There should be a legitimate reason for all work done and all work done should somehow move the athlete closer to the long-range training goal.

The body adapts to the stresses placed upon it—to a point. Recognition of the rhythmic training cycle of stress, rest and adaptation is one of the keys to success in the short run. Judicious use of training cycles will help to create a more solid foundation allowing one to successfully approach one's potential over the course of a career.

Vern Gambetta has stated that the concept of a "healthy athlete" is really an oxymoron, a contradiction of terms. With an understanding of training theory most would agree. But when one is armed with knowledge of training cycles, the critical importance of rest and a healthy respect for the preciousness of time athletic participation can prove to be a challenging and self-fulfilling pursuit when done by design.

Competition Travel Tips

One's packing expertise is directly proportional to one's travel frequency. If competition travel is a once in a season thing forethought and planning can make for an enjoyable experience as opposed to one marred by "stuff I forgot."

One of the great things about running is the opportunity of competition travel. Because of the universal participation in this sport the trips may be local, national or international. That being said there is some necessary planning that had better go into this travel so one's competitive efforts are optimized.

In truth two things need to be done when planning to travel to a competition. First one needs to establish a preparation ritual that becomes repeated event to event. It's strongly suggested creating a permanent list of all the things one needs to bring. One should also dedicate a travel bag that is solely used for travel and keep the list in the travel bag. That way when it comes to packing the whole process becomes almost mechanical.

The second point is to plan your travel bag over a three-week period. Admittedly this may seem like a long time but what it will do is allow you to critically think things through, things you need and things you won't. This should also help eliminate the gnawing feeling of "forgetting something" that can accompany a last-minute rush packing job.

It helps to lie out the clothing or other personal items in some systematic manner, for instance, items used from head to toe. This allows you to visualize what you need. Starting three weeks out allows you to modify your choices for practicality and comfort.

For local trips much of this planning will become second nature but when one makes a national or international trip forgetting something can be both inconvenient and expensive. For longer trips one thing to immediately figure out is how many time zones will be covered. For travel two to three time zones away there will not be much disruption in one's "body clock," but when one travels 6-12 time zones one can expect disrupted sleep patterns and meal schedules. Management and accommodation become the order of the day.

One thing that I have suggested is to wear two watches starting about three weeks out, one with the local time and a second watch with the destination time. This allows one to project how they will feel when they get to their destination. It also helps show that one's mindset is going to have to adapt. If one is accustomed to competing at 6pm "home time" and must travel to a different time zone that requires one to compete at 11pm "home time" there had better be some adaptation.

A final point regarding time, particularly with international travel is to familiarize yourself with a 24-hour clock or military time. Many countries do not use the AM/PM designation most Americans are used to and it would be both embarrassing and inexcusable to miss a competition because of mistaken time keeping.

Below are some other areas that should be considered when traveling:

Water—Always keep some bottled water within arm's reach. The excitement of travel with all the new sights and sounds can distract one from maintaining proper hydration. Bottled water also helps prevent So and So's Revenge. While most countries have sanitation standards similar to the United States it is not your job to experiment, it is to compete. Proper hydration also helps prevent constipation that will creep up on you if you don't maintain proper hydration.

Sleep—When traveling I suggest sleeping as much as possible, at every opportunity. This may not be how you spend your regular days but it will allow you to "bank" some sleep hours. Some may discount the idea of banking sleep, adding that you may arrive at your destination sluggish but you will not arrive overtired.

Once at your destination get on the local time schedule. Afternoon naps often lead to full-blown sleep sessions so initially resist them. Get up and walk around. Most people have more trouble adapting to time zone changes traveling to the East (i.e.—Europe, London, etc. from New York) than traveling West but when you travel over six time zones in any direction it will require some adaptation.

Food—Prior to one's competition keep it simple. While I fully encourage one to sample the local cuisine of different areas or countries it is best to do so after one has competed. Packing such things as peanut butter, crackers, cheese or some tuna fish may not adequately meet the required four food groups, but it will hold you over in a pinch. Other pre-packaged snacks such as power bars or granola bars are also a nice travel treat. Also consider taking some protein powder that can be mixed with the bottled water.

Competition bags—It is a good idea to have a separate competition bag similar to the travel bag with its use solely dedicated to competition items and a list of competition materials all its own. It never hurts to have a few extras in the bag such as safety pins and pliers for the last-minute emergency.

Clothes—With the proliferation of the Internet you can find out what the weather is in Timbuktu—now. This greatly helps your planning. Most people pack too much clothing. I've learned to pack three days' worth of clothing and then wash what you need. It may be only a sink wash with bar soap but with clothes semi-clean and dry one can soldier on. Pack an 8-10 foot length of rope for your clothesline.

What good clothes to bring is always an issue. What I have come to do is wear my good clothes as I travel. You can always get them cleaned or pressed when you arrive. Bringing an extra shirt or blouse can add much versatility to one's wardrobe.

Personal hygiene—While the contents of this portion of the travel bag will differ from men to women some common contents will greatly enhance one's transition to an unfamiliar location. Such staples as a toothbrush, toothpaste, hairbrush, razor and shave cream or gel, needle and thread, deodorant, nail clipper or nail file, band-aids, hand lotion, baby oil could all be purchased for less than $15. and will help normalize things at one's destination as quickly as possible.

Miscellaneous—Below are a number of things that have proven to be invaluable and don't take up much space or weigh much. One or two plastic containers with locking tops, a can opener, plastic zip lock bags, rubber bands, plastic ties, a game—preferably one that can be played with others like travel Scrabble or a dice or card game and finally two good books. I recommend lighter reading but also something you can "get into." Travel affords hours of down time and you'll be surprised that what you might normally read in a week or two will be completed in two to three days. The opportunity to share books will spur conversation that will ultimately make the whole experience more enjoyable.

While travel opportunities are certainly exciting, for many change can be intimidating. It therefore becomes of paramount importance to create as many common denominators of home as possible when one travels. The care and attention one puts into packing a travel bag will go a long way towards promoting a psychologically secure environment from which superlative efforts happen. It is a well-planned effort that ultimately makes all the time, effort and energy put into any endeavor all the more worthwhile.

VITAMIN C

As stated in the article this is a topic that few seem to agree on. Much of these comments are based on the work of Linus Pauling who won two Nobel prizes. He is considered one of the top scientists of all time, on the short list with the likes of Einstein, Newton and Pasteur. He practiced what he preached and lived an active life into his 90s. But I guess some would say he was just lucky.

Nowadays you can't see a news program or page through a newspaper without finding some tidbit by some guru on the latest health or diet aid. To complicate matters the next article or interview you come across probably contradicts the first one. The high protein v. high carbo diets are a recent example.

It is much the same with vitamins—"they are critical," "they make for expensive urine," "you don't need them if you eat right," and with 40% of America obese, who eats right? The arguments escalate to noise. What's a baby boomer to do?

Vitamins were the theoretical brainchild of a Polish biochemist named Funk. In the early 1900s the four biggest killer diseases in the world were scurvy (lack of vitamin C), pellagra (deficiency of niacin), beriberi (deficiency of thiamin) and rickets (deficiency of vitamin D). It was a leap of logic that Funk figured out that all these killers were related to the lack of something in the patient's food. Although it took years to substantiate Funk's theory time has proven he was correct.

What exactly is a vitamin? Vitamins are organic compounds (compounds recognized by the body) that cannot be made by the body and the absence of which creates disease. Most vitamins are also co-enzymes. A co-enzyme is a molecule that attaches to an enzyme, a larger molecule, that together create reactions and make things happen in our bodies. In a way vitamins are like hormones but they differ in that hormones are usually made in our body.

To date 41 vitamins have been identified that meet the above criteria. The most famous vitamin (another debatable subject) is vitamin C. Although few in the chorus would argue the necessity of vitamin C (to prevent scurvy) the harmony turns to noise once the how much, how often and what form questions begin to get asked.

Vitamin C is a water-soluble vitamin, meaning it breaks down in water. Water-soluble vitamins are not stored in the body. This is important in a vitamin's use because even in megadoses the side effects of water-soluble vitamins are not life threatening. In the case of vitamin C diarrhea is the tell-tale sign that one has had enough.

Why would anyone in the Land of Plenty need or want to take vitamin C? In the USA we are truly fortunate to have the best diets with the greatest variety of foods that humankind has ever seen. Think about it—you can walk into most large supermarkets, 24 hours a day and get kiwi's from New Zealand, pineapples from Hawaii or any other fruit or vegetable you desire.

But don't confuse our supermarkets with the Garden of

Eden. Just as we could eat good things (fresh fruits and vegetables) we have 24-hour access to the bad things too—the high fat, refined and processed foods of low to no nutritional value. The serpent of temptation resides in the aisle of chips and dips. Fats taste good and we wind up sacrificing nutritional value to our appetites. Ultimately, we pay for this indulgence later in life with degenerative diseases such as diabetes, heart disease and cancer.

Vitamin C is very important to a person who has an active lifestyle or competes. It is said that we take upwards of 10,000 steps a day. This places tremendous physical stress on the body. The foods we eat repair this micro trauma or repetitive stress of life, but if we don't eat well, living on refined and processed foods we create deficiencies in our bodies, we don't heal as well and we age more quickly (you can read that "die sooner").

Vitamin C is a vitamin that accomplishes many things in the body, not the least of which is to promote the healing and repair of collagen. Collagen is the substance that makes up the infrastructure of the cells, skin, bones, ligaments and cartilage of the body.

Vitamin C also functions as an anti-oxidant or free radical fighter. Free radicals are not reformed hippies from the 60s but rather atoms and molecules that pollute our body on a cellular level. Free radicals damage our immune systems, promote infection and de-generative diseases. Free radicals are formed from certain exposures (x-rays, environmental pollution, the sun's rays from the depletion of the ozone layer) and from the breakdown of stored fat that can be used for energy, the premise of the recent high protein diets.

Vitamin E is also a "free radical fighter" and interestingly works synergistically with vitamin C. A synergism is where one compound makes the other more effective—so it is a good idea if you are taking vitamin C to compliment it with vitamin E.

Vitamin C also plays a role in the growth and formation of some amino acids, the building blocks of proteins. Recent studies have also found vitamin C plays a role in neurotransmissions, aiding how thought signals are transferred through the body. Few would argue these points.

But once again the chorus begins to lose the verse when the experts are asked to comment on the validity of vitamin C's anti-cancer (it is an anti-oxidant), anti-viral or anti-cholesterol formation qualities. Personally, I think it will be only a matter of time until most healthcare providers arrive at these conclusions.

Vitamin C deficiencies are rare in industrialized countries (one needs only 9mg/day to prevent scurvy, a small baked potato has 45mg) with scurvy now a rare disease. More controversial diet claims suggest that alcoholics benefit from a nutritionally balanced diet high in vitamin C. Another claim is that children eat less candy with a balanced diet.

How do you know if you are getting enough vitamin C? Inadequate levels of vitamin C will produce bleeding gums, a tendency to bruise easily and hang nails. Although the minimum daily requirement (MDR) is 60mg that is really the bare minimum.

I recommend a baseline minimum of 3000mg daily. It doesn't really matter if the dose comes in 500mg or 1000mg tablets. You set your resolve, head for the local health food store and immediately are confused by your choices. Do you choose regular vitamin C or ester C? What is the difference?

Esterification is the addition of an alcohol molecule to the vitamin C molecule (like a co-enzyme to an enzyme) that slows down the breakdown of vitamin C. Why is this important? Ester C is a form of vitamin C that dissolves more slowly. Instead of having a spike of the vitamin levels soon after ingestion of the pill ester C's breakdown is more gradual offering a constant level of vitamin over a 6-8 hour period.

Pregnant women should not take more than 5000mg of vitamin C a day or the newborn may come to suffer from rebound scurvy soon after birth. If colds and flus seem impending one can use a "vitamin C flush" of 1000mg of vitamin C an hour until diarrhea sets in. Diarrhea is the signal one has had enough. Consult a healthcare practitioner before embarking on any personal experiments.

Just as Funk had theorized 100 years ago many of the diseases we succumb to today are the result of poor food selection and long term unhealthy eating habits. While vitamin C is not the "magic bullet" it certainly has health benefits that far outweigh its cost. For healthy, active individuals, vitamin C plays a vital role in the tissue repair and general health, well being and enjoyment of our chosen recreational activities.

When I was a Child

We all go through the same phases of life. Some people handle it more successfully than others. Change can be intimidating but it also can be planned for. We often forget what it was like being a child athlete evolving into an adolescent athlete. For those who made the transition much of this article will make sense. For those that did not make the transition, they'll probably never see this article.

There is a line in the Bible that goes, "When I was a child I thought like a child." It goes on and essentially references how change is a critical factor in our personal development as we transition through the phases of life.

In one's "athletic life" there are also changes that we all master with different levels of success. I have written before on the three general stages an athlete progresses through—fun, commitment and performance based efforts, but even a general awareness of these only minimally prepares one to make the transitions.

Improvement necessitates change. This statement has almost become a cliché. Einstein is credited with stating that one form of insanity is to repeat the same procedures again and again without change and expect to get a different result. To produce a different result necessitates changing one's approach, which for most is easier said than done.

If all things only grow once life truly becomes a "one shot deal." To realize our true potential, our growth, our development does not tolerate significant missteps. What complicates this whole process is that the vast majority of people live life with a forward view of about 200 yards. A runner will get that. It is about 30 seconds if you are moving fast and maybe two minutes if you're walking. What happens past that 200 yards depends on a plan, on a belief in the plan and the faith that it can/will happen. But if one's attention span is the length of a sound bite you can expect about as much future planning and directional thought as that of a windblown plastic bag.

The preferred and hopefully for many, the initial exposure to sport was fun, it was like play. This is where early attempts to organize children's sports often fall short, especially in activities where the child cannot fathom the rules of the game. It only produces a form of chaos with little lasting learning value.

And chaos, a lack of structure, with little learned presents a poor foundation for future reference, especially for a child. If there is no plan or they fail to see a plan (planned development) the default tendency will be to assume things will be done this way, always, with little attention to design. Using their only point of reference they "think like a child."

But nothing stays the same. Growth of the body involves weight and height changes, new thought patterns and deeper understandings, taste and preferences changes that can all present with their own set of challenges.

Interestingly one of the most stunning changes for the young athlete is muscle soreness. A child in the fun/play stage rarely gets sore. They are really not trained, they are active until they tire and then they rest. It is a simple participation formula.

Organized competition, with clearly defined quarters, periods or distances presents a new set of "rules" that participation mandates. Other factors such as one's will to win or succeed can provide the impetus to push past the point of fatigue, to give that extra 10% to succeed. And the price to be paid can be sore muscles.

But the child, thinking like a child, does not anticipate this. There is nothing in their past reference for this "new" situation. And for some this change, this new reality is more than they have bargained for. It becomes easier to back off, take the path of least resistance. One of the reasons often sited why children quit sport as they become adolescents is that it is no longer "fun." While the pain may be temporary and the pride a participation forever, the pain part is never fun.

Another big change the adolescent athlete must adopt is the simple warm-up and warm down. To an experienced adult this is a no-brainer. It is just something one does, but again in their distant past this habit was added to one's daily workouts and competition prep. The warm-up and warm down become ritualized habits that have health and performance implications; but again, once upon a time there was a day when this was a new behavior, a change that the athlete adopted whether they did so willingly or with some degree of trepidation.

This ability to handle change might be seen as the maturing process. Who would disagree with this? For one, I can think of the "terminally immature." These individuals, set in their ways, the ways of a child with childish thinking, most would see as an impediment to their progress.

While it is possible these people still may achieve a

degree of accomplishment it usually is at great cost. The sporting news and Internet weekly chronicle the missteps of the American celebrity athlete. While to the average/sane/normal reader (if there such a person) the actions and behaviors of said athlete may prove to be equally baffling/entertaining/troubling. And note that these observations are done from afar. No doubt these behaviors are viewed differently from the perspective of a coach, administrator or teammate. This "me first—the heck with you" thought can lose games, ruin seasons and prematurely end careers.

The hindsight of a 20-something and beyond of childhood is that of an idyllic time oftentimes forgetting the tremendous personal changes and challenges of new and different things.

A common sentiment many people share is that upon return to a childhood home or school reunion is the vague feeling of how small everything is. In the interceding years one has grown physically and often one's world has expanded so that what was once new and intimidating has been reduced to something old and familiar.

Adolescence is a time of growth physically, emotionally, even spiritually. An understanding and developing appreciation for this time of growth can be fostered with the use of appropriate role models and progressive goal setting that will forecast the changes and challenges that are coming.

Change can be intimidating but with attention to fundamental development it can be both negotiated and managed successfully so that the perspective on one's career, at the end of the road, is that of satisfaction with one's efforts as opposed to the feeling that the lack thereof is someone else's fault.

The 10 Day Rule

There are immediate consequences for a superlative effort. The motivated athlete or coach does a great job of creating the superlative performance but can lose "control" when they let the motivation of that superlative effort dictate planning for the next training cycle. Rest and recovery are the order of the day.

When you are young and just getting started in sports, particularly a sport like running it is easy to get lulled into a false sense that improvements will follow a straight-line path from race to race forever or at least to the next Olympics, whichever comes first.

The reality check for most athletes is when the personal bests reach a "peak." In truth a peak is a nebulous concept to a newbie where the next PR correlates well with the next competitive effort. To a vet the peak represents the time of a season or year where all the hard work, hopes and directed dreams converge for that one special moment.

But that special moment can create problems in itself. Intoxicating thoughts of continued breakthroughs, grandeur, fame and fortune goad one to forge ahead with renewed effort and little regard for one's personal health.

For some this unchecked motivation can be as destructive as it is productive. Most readers with any experience can point to a season or career best that was followed in short order by an unplanned illness or injury that left one frustrated and confused as to what went wrong and asking—why did it have to happen now?

Personal bests require the body to take a leap into uncharted territory and can be very stressful for the body. The personal best requires the body to do something it has never done before. There is an overreaching situation that even with months or years of training the body is not prepared for the stress. The body has been physically shocked—in a true sense and needs time to regroup.

Most physiology books detail the prodromal or latency period an organ or body system needs to return to normal following a bout of exercise (Chart 2). We intuitively know this. The body needs special rest after the shock of a personal best. Most runners seem to only get this wisdom through trial and error. The errors can be career costly.

Chart 2 – Recovery Times of Body Systems	
Heart rate	20-60 minutes
Cellular nutrients	4-6 hours
Proteins	12-24 hours
Fats, vitamins, enzymes	24+ hours
Muscular system	24-48 hours
Strength	48-72 hours
Anaerobic lactate system	48 hours
Maximal aerobic system	48-56 hours
Aerobic endurance	48-56 hours
Central nervous system	7x muscular system
(adapted from Bompa, Platonov '88)	

Heart rate returns to normal after 20-60 minutes. Of particular note is that the muscular system requires 24-48 hours to recover. Note that the nervous system takes 7x that of the muscular system. The systemic shock of a superlative effort is not simply resolved with a warm meal and a good night's sleep.

Traditionally I have always taught that for every 5 minutes raced one needs one day of recovery. That works well for a 40-minute 10K personal record but what is the recovery rule for a personal best in the mile or the bench press for that matter?

The first time I heard of the 10 Day Rule I was reading a book by sprint coach Charlie Francis. He noted that following the world class personal best he routinely "rested" his athletes 10 days. Remember that the nervous system takes seven times as long as the muscular system to recover. The accepted time for the muscle recovery is 24-48 hours. Seven times the middle 36 hours is 252 hours or 10.5 days. The concept of rest may need some explaining.

Rest as used here is really a conscientious effort at allowing the body, including the organs, systems, nutrient, hormone and enzyme levels adequate time to normalize and recover to a higher state of fitness. A more accurate term to describe this period may be "aggressive rest" where one moderately exercises but more importantly includes close attention to other activities that promote healing and recovery in the body.

Maximal use is always abuse. Many athletes engage in competition with the mistaken concept that what they are doing solely benefits the body. While the exercise and fitness levels one attains from athletic participation cannot be disputed overuse syndromes and physiologic illnesses are also an ever-present possibility.

The reality of competition schedules, training philosophies, team commitments, coaching or lack of personal self discipline can individually and or collectively combine to create an athletic experience that falls short of the ideal. Efforts to squeeze in 10 days worth of what might be seen as wasted time or questionable efforts, especially during a time of high fitness might seem ridiculous.

It is like driving a hot rod in neutral—all you can do is

rev the engine and coast. The work you are doing is not "getting you anywhere." With a short-term view you are right. But what this rest or coasting period is doing is allowing the body to regroup and rebuild and adapt to a higher state of fitness required for the next step.

For a motivated athlete this can be a difficult concept to swallow—especially the first time you hear it. It doesn't make sense. Competition is all about striking while the iron is hot. But we've all seen sprinters do this countless times. Once free of the field in a trial or semi they motor down and ease across the finish line. To the uninformed fan the sprinter is hot-dogging it. The wise sprinter has exerted his or her dominance and wisely saves energy for the race that really counts.

For most athletes the personal best represents a high-water mark in their career. The day or the moment can be proudly recounted for years afterwards. Unfortunately for many others their career is summarized with a sense of regret for the race or competition that never happened because some unplanned injury that unexpectedly happened when everything else was going right.

A recent study found that 48% of participants in individual sports were over trained, did too much work too often. The motivation of the individual drove them past the point of fatigue to a state that they could not recover from. The causes may be many from poor coaching to peer pressure to personal irresponsibility, but the result remains the same—conversations of lament replace those of "I did." Awareness and attention to the 10 Day Rule will offer some direction that mixed with patience and a long-term plan for development will grant one the opportunity of greater things.

Training Maxims

We live in a sound bite world, daily we are inundated with catchy slogans that urge us to buy this or that. It happens in running too. There are bumper stickers and t-shirt slogans that can succinctly summarize our hopes and desires. But the best maxims are the ones that bring us to action.

A maxim is a pithy statement that the dictionary defines as a "concise rule of conduct." And while that may allow the maximist to get a little preachy the lesson hinges on the intent.

Detailed below are a series of training maxims that concisely speak to things one should (and shouldn't) do to maximize athletic performance. While I doubt most will agree with every saying I am confident any coach, athlete, teacher or parent will find more wheat than chaff.

The limiting factor in athletic performance is not enough time. From start to finish (or at least significant decline) most athletic careers last 10-12 years. Some master competitors may go on forever, but improved performance does not. This underscores the import of planned training and recovery efforts in order to optimize one's potential. Poor planning, a reckless lifestyle and haphazard efforts produce haphazard results. Time is of the essence.

Train with intention. If one's goal is improvement should not all one's efforts be directed to that end? Therefore, one needs to critically evaluate the various components of a training plan (interval training, strength work, pre-hab efforts, biomotor skill development, etc.) to see if they are aiding or hindering one's training goals. Lifestyle also comes into play, therefore living with intention is a good idea too. This involves knowledge and forethought and the sense to reevaluate as necessary. Mindlessness has no focus. Don't just do it.

Speed is a function of strength. If one's goal is to run fast one needs to be strong. All top-level sprinters are powerful people. Power is defined as a combination of speed and strength. While various methods to strengthen the legs can be used (weights, hiking, long slow distance) strengthening the prime movers (gluts, quads, TFL, hamstrings, gastric/soleus) is critical if one is to run faster. Weight training with a progressive overload is the safest and simplest way.

Psychological strength comes from psychological security. The "home court advantage" happens because prior to (and during) a competitive event one knows the venue, the registration procedures, travel times, and such simple creature comforts as where the water fountains and bathrooms are. The elimination of "surprises" that alter one's competitive focus need to me minimized through planning and trouble shooting before the big day.

The limiting factor in athletic performance is energy/nutrition. Life is an endurance sport. The quality and length of our lives is directly affected by the quality of the food we ingest. In a competitive situation the depletion of the body's energy stores ("hitting the wall") has taken on mythic qualities. The expressions of speed, strength or endurance all hinge in part, on the fuel in the tank, our nutritional stockpile.

Nothing goes in your mouth by accident. The exception to this rule might be a bug or bee but past that—let's get real, Twinkies, drugs, alcohol or "more than enough" are the results of our willpower or lack thereof. Temptation can be answered by critically evaluating the object of one's desire and asking, "What part of my body do I want this to become?"

You are what you eat. How could this not be true? High salt, high sugar, processed foods loaded with trans-fats do little for the body other than taste good and temporarily satisfy hunger. These fillers are empty calories that cannot be built upon. In the early days of computer programming there was a saying "garbage in—garbage out" and everyone came to know what that meant. It works for food too.

Vitamin supplementation is meant to enhance food, not replace it. In America we are enamored with pills. The pharmaceutical industry has a pill for every stage of one's life, for problems real and imagined. There is a tendency to believe that pills cure all ills. Processed foods, genetically engineered grains from heavily fertilized, devitalized ground produces devitalized foods. Vitamin supplementation can help make-up for nutritional short falls. But one must still start with the highest quality fruits, vegetables and protein sources available.

Insecurity over prepares. Many people mistakenly equate "extra effort" with success. Whether it is one more set or rep or mile they reason that this extra effort is what will ultimately distinguish them from the competition. As often as not this extra effort leads to an overtraining situation, whether it is an illness or injury in the short run or significant breakdown and shortened career in the long run. This underscores the "train with intention" maxim. And if you live and die by the thought "good enough is never enough"—get some help.

Process precedes outcome. For the musician to complete a musical piece they must complete a series of notes (or combinations of notes) in sequence. One sound follows another. When this is done with timing and coordination music is produced. From the unskilled we get noise. For an athlete to solely focus on the end goal without attention to perfection of the daily steps blurs focus of the here and now. Goals may offer direction, but it is what one does at this moment that one can control. If the daily process is learned and done correctly a successful outcome will follow.

Practice what you can, not what you can't. If I were to tell you that I could change a Cadillac into a Rolls Royce by driving it faster, you'd laugh at me. For that transformation to take place you'd have to change and improve the parts. To train physically as a four-minute miler when you are running 4:20s will only lead to frustration and injury. An honest evaluation of one's current fitness level is necessary. Perfect that process and then shoot for an incremental improvement. Success more often comes by approximation than with a fantastic leap.

Never create doubt. Doubt is a cancer of the mind. One of the things that distinguish successful athletes from the run of the mill ones is the unshakable belief that a goal can be accomplished. Part of that belief is the role the coach and important others (teammates, parents, teachers, etc.) play in creating an, "I can do this," environment. Necessarily part of this environment is the presentation or creation of challenges that (through process) are met and accomplished. This creates an inventory of success and a mindset on the part of the athlete that with preparation and diligent application the challenges can be successfully met. If sarcasm, cynicism and cutting remarks are mixed with unrealistic goals success or failure will be left to chance. When the first thought one faced with a challenge is, "I can do this," the battle is more than half won.

When training children—don't fatigue the system. For the child there is a fine line between growth and development and training and competition. While they both can happen simultaneously should one pair dominate it is to the detriment of the other. The reason one cannot do both is due to the limited energy reserves of the body. Childhood and adolescence are times that place significant energy demands on the body due to growth. If a child is highly trained or over competed energies that would go towards growth and development are shunted towards competitive survival. Allowing the child to transition through periods of fun (ages 6-11), commitment (ages 12-17) and performance (18+) offer a more natural progression that roughly parallels the mental and physical development stages to maturity. What constitutes system fatigue? Tudor Bompa has recommended 65% efforts, but that can be difficult to quantify. A simple clue to early fatigue is when the laughing stops and the hands go on the knees—workout done.

All things only grow once. Therefore, some believe, you should train the child hard from the start, let them get used to it and they will grow with it. This didn't work with the child labor tragedies of the 1800s so why would it work with athletic competition? What this maxim speaks to is the necessity of engraining fundamentals. These fundamentals could be movement patterns, thought patterns or problem-solving skills. Engrained problem-solving skills, behaviors and attitudes along with a progressive history of successfully meeting challenges creates within the young athlete an inventory of knowledge, skills and abilities that can be developed as one moves through the higher levels of competition. This value system, developed early on, creates a self-support system when the inevitable setbacks, failures and frustrations of life stymie one's efforts. It is the strength of this value system that determines whether the obstacle is a stumbling block or a steppingstone.

The body adapts to the stresses placed upon it. This statement is true to a point. If the stress the body faces is gradual and progressive the body will react by adapting with increased speed, strength or endurance. It becomes important that the training be focused to the task demands of the event or sport. To train a marathoner's vertical jumping ability would be a waste of time just as it would be wasted time to train a high jumper's ability to run a marathon. But with too much focused training without adequate recovery time the body will not adapt to training and overtraining, illness or injury will result. At the higher levels of training this is a fine line.

Train movements, not muscles. This is a maxim attributed to training theorist Tudor Bompa. All sporting activities are a sequence of multiple movements with the timing and coordination of these movements critical for efficient technical execution, energy efficient movements and refinement of force application. Because of this resistance training (including weight training, medicine ball work, kettle bells, etc.) is most fruitful when the whole body, or at least major portions of the body are trained mimicking the movements of the technique or sport.

Bodybuilding exercises (biceps curls, seated leg extensions, calf raises, etc.) may help with general fitness and develop aesthetic appeal but these isolated movements usually transfer poorly to a "whole action" like running, throwing or playing a position on a team.

The dynamic stabilizers are the exception to this rule. Dynamic stabilizers are muscles that stabilize joint complexes as we move. The glut medius, psoas, adductor group or posterior tibialis of the foreleg would be examples. These muscles warrant special attention, either pre-hab work or when injured, rehab work so they can successfully meet the demands they may face. Training movements, not muscles is a maxim true 80-90% of the time.

Flexibility should be optimized, not maximized. Flexibility is the only noncompetitive biomotor skill. The problem with becoming too flexible is that it dampens the neuromuscular response of the body, which is another way of saying it dampens the body's speed and reaction time. Different activities will require different levels of flexibility, the hurdler versus the marathoner, yet both could become too flexible for their event. Freedom of range of motion within the technical demands of an activity is the goal; improvements past that point are wasted time and non-productive.

All growth and development comes while resting. If one were to run a hard 400m, rest 15 seconds and try it again—what would be the benefit? Probably very little. The recovery time was too short. In a competitive training situation, one's recovery time should be as closely monitored as one's training. In fact, there is a sub-maxim here—recover as hard as you train. When this process is carefully monitored optimal growth and development will result. To neglect, ignore or otherwise minimize the importance of adequate recovery courts illness, injury and systemic breakdown.

Maximal use is always abuse. Rich Phaigh, a massage therapist for Athletics West is credited with this statement. When one starts to move faster than 95% effort the coordination of the body starts to unravel. One needs to accept the fact that speed and speed actions represent the ultimate coordination of the body. Coordination is a pattern and maximal effort is by its very nature something that has not been done before, it is a new experience by the body and because the performance is "new" there is no pattern for it. The problem is that the body attempts to use old patterns to perform new actions that are uncoordinated and at least minimally damaging to the body, even though this is on a microscopic level. But repeated time and time again without proper recovery methods these microscopic injuries accumulate. The replacement scar tissue that forms, tears more easily and can lead to more serious, possibly career-ending injury. Age 35 seems to be the age where the "maximal use" of a career is no longer tolerated by the body. Coincidentally that is roughly the age most high-level careers come to an end.

Fatigue is a defense mechanism of the body. When a car's energy system (gasoline) is depleted it stops. The depletion of energy stores in the body due to hard work, what marathoners call "hitting the wall" signals the end of high intensity effort. When you are done, you're done. Take the hint, rest up and return to perform another day.

Training to failure is training to fail. In America our mythic sports heroes always give 110%. But do they really? Once fatigue has set in and there is a technique breakdown (rigor mortis, poorly controlled or uncoordinated movements) one is no longer training patterns that clarify neuromuscular response, coordinate force application or maximize body efficiency. Practicing with technical breakdown is practicing things one does not want to duplicate in a performance effort and is often one step away from injury. Perfect practice makes perfect. Sometimes good enough is good enough. Let it go at that.

People are 80% water and water always takes the easiest course. An obsessive-compulsive person has it their way all day, everyday and they drive themselves and everybody else crazy. A person who works at 80% efficiency rate is seen as highly organized and somebody who can "get things done." The price of perfection is prohibitive. The difference between perfect and done is perfect is never done.

I can do this. This is sports psychology in four words. If one's mindset when facing a challenge or obstacle is in this positive direction the likelihood of success is greatly enhanced. Faith, confidence, belief and affirmative action are all implied with this simple statement.

Basic body fitness begins at the core. The muscular stability of the abdomen and core muscles is critical for anyone wishing to run, jump or throw in a competitive circumstance. Planks, side planks, sit-ups and push-ups are simple exercises to get one started.

Training at the performance level is not a natural or healthy thing to do to your body. If you were an "average" person cruising the aisles of a local supermarket how apt would you be to run a marathon? Or perform a maximal bench press? Or run 10x400m in 80 seconds? Or do depth jumps or a plyometric routine? Not very likely. Maximal use is always abuse. Highly competitive efforts place abnormal stresses on the body. Over the course of time this damage accumulates with varying degrees of injury or illness. It is important one see this distinction between fitness and performance-based efforts where one strives for a personal best. The fitness activities can be used to build up the body. Performance based efforts create a situation where damage to the body is the result of the maximal effort which underscores the importance of recovery effort.

Children are not little adults. One of the most difficult things I have ever had to write was the distance running curriculum for the USATF Youth Level II Coaching Education Program. I researched all the great distance coaches, in the world, and not one had anything to say about coaching the child distance runner. Ultimately, I came up with four recommendations—keep it simple, keep it short, keep it fun and keep it fast. For the adult distance runner this would produce limited results, but who really cares about the performance results of a child? The performance marks a 10-year-old makes give little indication of future potential. Doubt this? Google the American or World Records for 10-year-olds in the mile, 5k, 10k, half-marathon and marathon. Not one of these kids had any success as an adult if they even continued to run that long.

Fundamental movement patterns, personal self-discipline, personal responsibility, a rudimentary idea of what practice is about and how to work with others are noble goals for entry level programs—for any sport. Children are not little adults—don't train them that way. Keep it simple, keep it short, keep it fast and keep it fun.

Either pre-hab or rehab. Pre-hab is a series of movement drills done at the beginning of a workout session. Pre-hab efforts could be part of a dynamic warm-up that could include things such as foot drills, skipping, high knees, etc. The point of pre-hab is to tone or condition the general body or focal areas of the body for the stresses one faces in running, jumping or throwing.

Rehab efforts are focused activities necessary to repair a breakdown of a specific body part, usually due to overuse. The problem with rehab efforts is that they require a disruption in the long-term training schedule. They represent down time, a holding pattern of no improvement. This time becomes problematic in that weeks, months or even years spent in this state steal time that could be used for development of one's potential. While rehab is critical to the ill or injured athlete it results from poor training plan design and in the grand scheme is wasted effort.

The Bijou Mile

This was a great race. It was one of the few times all the best runners in the area would come together. We had a schedule that clicked like clockwork and produced some great performances that people still talk about almost 30 years later.

The battery to my large digital clock had crapped out. I was on my way to Battery World in Syracuse to get it replaced. On the drive I figured this was the third time since I owned the clock I had to get the battery replaced. And then I realized I bought the clock over 30 years ago. How time flies.

I bought the clock along with a ladder system finish line structure for the first Bijou Mile. For those new to the area the Bijou Mile was a one mile run down Broadway in Saratoga Springs. Those were the days when road miles were a new wrinkle to road racing. In the seven years we ran the race it was one of the fixtures of the Capital District's racing schedule.

The original plan for the Bijou Mile was to run a series of four races over the course of the summer. But I needed a sponsor first. Downtown Saratoga had a few possibilities. The problem was getting the finish line to end in front of the establishment which in turn affected where the start line would be up North Broadway. If we finished too close to the Post Office we'd have to settle for a narrow start up near Skidmore College.

Finishing in front of the Bijou Bar was just right. But I didn't think the management would go for it. The Bijou wasn't quite a biker bar but the women in there had tattoos before women had tattoos.

I met Ralph Spillinger, the Bijou owner and gave him my pitch. Road race, ends in front of your place, we video the race, show it after the race on your TV's, big crowd, big night for you. Back in 1985 video was still a "new" technology. Being able to see yourself on TV would be a novelty. We could plan a beer special, have the awards ceremony on the back stage, make a night of it.

Ralph was not a runner. He owned the Bijou and played in a band called The Students. They were a hot local group, had a large following and one of the members, Dave Twarog, was a good local runner. Ralph gave my pitch a moment's thought and said, "Yes."

Now all I needed was the OK from the City. For that I was directed to the Director of Public Safety, Chief Cole. My mother's family was from Saratoga and we spent every summer of my childhood there. More specifically I spent every waking moment at the Wright Street Gate of the Saratoga Race Track.

It all started with Lucky Pencils as a 5-year-old. Then came tip sheets, club house passes, used racing forms and programs, handing out flyers, finding lost cars—if we could turn a buck on it, we did it. Broadway Pete, Clocker Wilson, the guys who rented chairs, "taxi-car-taxi" guys, professional gamblers, hookers and homeless hangers-on, Wright Street had them all. And the man who kept the lid on the pot was Sgt. Cole.

Sgt. Cole rode a tricycle motorcycle. Before you think

that was a point of ridicule, think again. At 6'4" and over 300 pounds he rumbled down Wright St. like Ben-Hur in a Roman chariot. If there was anything that was not supposed to be happening, it stopped immediately. To get chased was one thing, to get caught led to banishment, an expensive possibility.

I sat in Cole's outer office convinced he would remember me, and not in a good way. The ability to run fast served me well but now there was nowhere to run. I formally introduced myself and explained my plan. I mentioned that the Bijou was on board and noted all my race management experiences throughout the Capital District and then shut up.

Chief Cole's first words were, "I don't want to do this." His concern was the traffic congestion it would cause. I assured him, start to finish, it would be over in one-hour. He objected to the four Friday nights, particularly during Track season. I floated the compromise of doing it just one Friday night before the Track season got underway. I told him if the event was a bust, I wouldn't be back. He was silent.

"I guess we could do this one time," he said.

My heart leapt and then the work began. The course was measured, the Saratoga Stryders were hired to do traffic control. Saratoga Video was contracted to do the video of the race. Officer Harry Redgrave, a childhood neighbor, was assigned to coordinate the race with me. On The Road's race crew included Matt Jones and Mike Lochner with wives Cathy Jones and Laurie Lochner hired to handle registration duties. All we needed was some runners.

And we got runners. Through flyers at the Colonie Summer Meets, Empire State Games trials and word of mouth we got runners. The first year we ran a men's and women's divisions. The races drew about 40 and 20 runners each. The lead-up to the race went smoothly. My only miscalculation was the race start time.

I wanted to capitalize on the downtown night life so I figured running the races at 8:45pm and 9:00pm would be a good idea. While we had a well-lit finish area, the start was in the dark. At 8:45 the light for the women was two shades darker than dusk. At 9:00pm the start for the men was pitch black.

As I gave the guys the obligatory pre-race directions a voice from the abyss cried, "Which way do we run?" It was a good question.

North Broadway looked like a dark tunnel with the red and white car lights 1000 yards away. All I could say was— "See those lights?"

Remember, 1985 pre-dates all cell phones. Even walkie-talkies did not carry for a mile. To time the race we had to start the watches with the gun shot and somehow beat the runners to the finish line. Bicycles were the obvious answer and that is what we wound up using for the 400/800 splits. The lead police vehicle had an open seat so that is what we used to get the watches to the finish.

With the gun shot the police car sped away. And I mean sped. Downtown Saratoga has a different vibe when you are traveling down Broadway at 60+ miles per hour. All the traffic was stopped and 45-50 seconds later we'd slow to the finish line, cue the video guy, set the overhead clock and wait for the runners.

The first year no one knew what to expect. The downhill was steep enough to give everyone a boost but not so much that one felt like losing control. Former UNH star Kathy Brandell from Plattsburgh began the evening with a

4:46.3 effort. The guys hit the 400 in 53 with no idea if that was fortuitous or the prelude to a disaster. Merrick Jones, a former Syracuse star, outlasted what would be the Bijou Mile's deepest field, narrowly missing the 4-minute mile with a 4:00.5 time. Seventh place was a 4:07.9.

The races ended, the runners were exhausted but pumped. Virtually everyone got a lifetime PR by 10-12 seconds. The video worked to perfection and all that was left to do was the clean-up. And then the fire siren went off.

In all my planning for the worst-case scenarios, a fire call was right up there with a car accident. The Saratoga Fire Station is on Lake Avenue about 200 yards from the Post Office. As the fire engines pulled out of the station I could see their lights reflected on City Hall. I was praying they would continue straight up Church Street away from us. No luck. They turned south, down Broadway, straight for us.

Remember I had invested $3000 in a finish line structure and clock and we had the whole street blocked off in front of the Bijou. This was not going to have a happy ending if we just stood still. The crowd went quiet. I looked at Matt Jones and we instinctively moved in unison as we pivoted the whole finish line structure 90 degrees to allow the fire trucks to zoom through. I laughed a nervous laugh at the close call. The crowd gave us a standing ovation.

We got some good press, the runners got lifetime PR's and even the police were psyched to be part of this event. In my review meeting with Chief Cole he noted that his "reports" came back positive and we were given the OK for a year two.

The Bijou Mile ran for six more years. It became a summer race fixture strategically placed between Empire

State Games Trials and Finals. Merrick Jones came back three years later to run the first sub-four-minute mile in upstate New York. In the seven years the race was held we had over 35 ESG champions compete in all the divisions.

As word spread we would get runners from Buffalo to Maine, from Pennsylvania, Philly and South Jersey. We were one of the first races to allow wheelchairs with guys scooting the mile in 3:23. Eventually the program was expanded to nine races that were run over 75 minutes. Through juggling the schedule and using staggered starts we were able to have a continuous stream of finishers all recorded by Saratoga Video.

In all the years the Saratoga Police were instrumental in making the race a success. Yearly we recognized local people and groups who made contributions. If you are ever in the Saratoga Police Station you can see a Bijou Mile plaque behind the registration desk.

Winners and placers for both the men and women's races reads like a who's who of area running greatness. Queenbury's Quinten Howe eventually set the men's record with a 3:56 in the final Bijou Mile. Saratoga's Cheri Goddard was a multiple time winner in both the open and high school divisions holding the records in both. Colonie's Todd Orvis held the high school mile record while Bill Robinson and Pennsylvania's John Serro share the masters record at 4:13.0.

As fame of the race spread Bijou Mile winners were eventually invited to run the 5th Avenue Mile held each fall in New York City. While the reluctance of that race's organizers was initially vexing, the success of our master and high school division winners made the Bijou Mile a legitimate proving ground for the NYC race.

Politics, politics and politics eventually ended the race.

Chief Cole was sympathetic and supportive to the end but to the disappointment of many the race disappeared in the summer of 1992. The Bijou moved on and only the memories remain. But I'm willing to bet that if you do run into somebody who ran the race their lasting memory will be—"The Bijou Mile, yeah, I got my mile PR there."

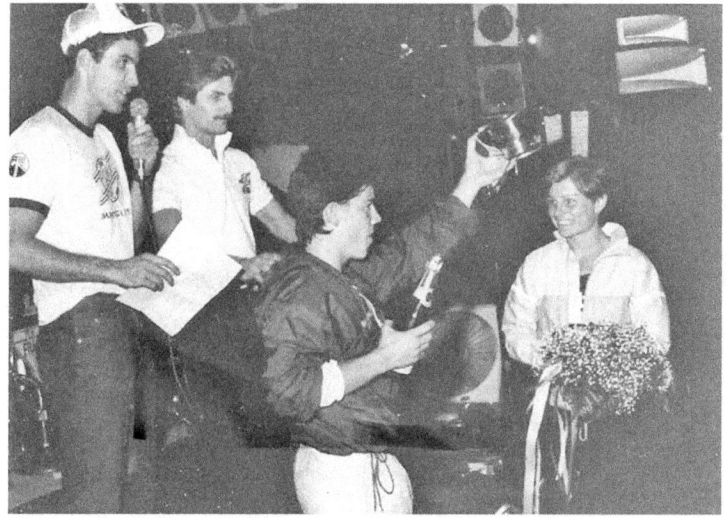

(Left to right) Russ Ebbets, Gary Leone, Bijou manager, 1st Annual Bijou Mile Champions (1985) Merrick Jones and Kathy Brandell

Author's Note

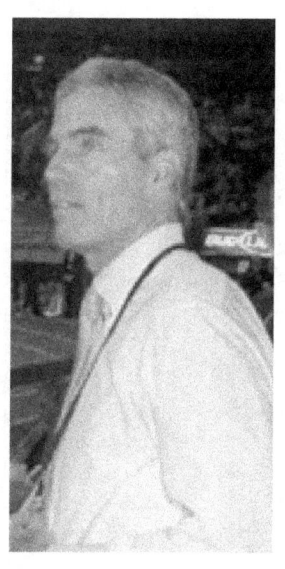

Russ Ebbets has taught in the USATF Coaching Education for over 35 years, speaking at Level 1, 2 and 3 schools and the High Performance Summits on distance running.

He has served as the US National Team chiropractor to three IAAF World Championships. His documentation and standards of care for on-site sports chiropractic have been adopted nationally. He has directed complimentary chiropractic care at over 250 events, 25 national championships and overseen the treatment of some 15,000 athletes at events ranging from local 5k's to Friehofer's *Run for Women*, Utica's *Boilermaker* and the *Millrose Games* at Madison Square Garden.

Since 1999 he has been editor of *Track Coach*, the technical journal of USATF. *Track Coach* enjoys a worldwide circulation and is seen as one of the leading training journals of the sport. Ebbets has lectured throughout the US, in Canada, Scandinavia and the Caribbean. Since the fall of 1983 he has contributed regularly to *Pace Setter Magazine* with his *Off The Road* column. Ultimately, he has proved Bill Reynolds right, one thing has led to another.

CPSIA information can be obtained
at www.ICGtesting.com
Printed in the USA
BVHW040814171219
566784BV00007B/7/P